Being Well (Even When You're Sick)

being well
(even when you're sick)

Mindfulness Practices
for People with Cancer
and Other Serious Illnesses

• • • • • • • • • •

Elana Rosenbaum

Foreword by Jon Kabat-Zinn

Shambhala
Boston & London
2012

Shambhala Publications, Inc.
Horticultural Hall
300 Massachusetts Avenue
Boston, Massachusetts 02115
www.shambhala.com

9 8 7 6 5 4 3 2 1

First Edition

Printed in the United States of America

♾This edition is printed on acid-free paper that meets the American National
Standards Institute Z39.48 Standard.
♻This book is printed on 30% postconsumer recycled paper. For more infor-
mation please visit www.shambhala.com.

Distributed in the United States by Random House, Inc.,
and in Canada by Random House of Canada Ltd

LIBRARY OF CONGRESS CATALOGING-IN-PUBLICATION DATA
Rosenbaum, Elana.
Being well (even when you're sick): mindfulness practices for people with can-
cer and other serious illnesses / Elana Rosenbaum; foreword by Jon Kabat-Zinn.
p.   cm.
Includes bibliographical references and index.
ISBN 978-1-61180-000-5 (pbk.)
1. Health—Psychological aspects. 2. Mind and body. 3. Self-care, Health. 4.
Alternative medicine. I. Title.
RA776.5.R673 2012
613—dc23
2011042584

Contents

Foreword

No one seeks such a rude awakening . . . a cancer diagnosis that threatens everything one most cherishes. When the full catastrophe of the human condition rears its head in our lives and underscores our ineluctable frailty, we can easily lose hope and all perspective. It is virtually inevitable to some degree, before other elements reenter the picture and restore a wider strategy of approach and a willingness to see the potential workability of even such unwanted news. As an aid in that coming to terms with what most needs facing and making room for—comes this book and its accompanying guided mindfulness and compassion practices. Elana Rosenbaum balances the enormity of what befalls us when we fall ill with an equally enormous proposition, namely that we can discover that we can also be well, and profoundly well at that, right in the same moment.

She herself is a living example of it, almost twenty years after an initial diagnosis of lymphoma, a harrowing yet life-saving stem cell transplantation procedure, and later, several recurrences. She speaks from the enormity of that unwanted and rending yet also ennobling apprenticeship. She also speaks with the modest grace and deeply rooted authenticity of someone whose work for a very long time has been both as an MBSR teacher and a mindfulness-informed psychotherapist working primarily with people with cancer.

Elana is a dynamo of a human being. She was when I first met her, and she is now as well, although older and perhaps more measured in the wake of her cancer. She is always using her energies and her skill to help others. I have known her for a long time. You might say we grew up together as we taught the MBSR program in the Stress Reduction Clinic and the Center for Mindfulness at the University of Massachusetts Medical School and UMass Memorial Hospital. But I met her even before the beginning of MBSR, when she was working as a psychotherapist at the Fallon Clinic, next door to the Medical Center, and would come over to take my yoga class each week. Some days, she drove me to Worcester, since we both lived in the Cambridge area. She became one of the first teachers of MBSR—and she has been teaching it ever since.

Elana defies all description, although, as you will see when you read the book, "the little engine who could," which she herself evokes, is not an inappropriate descriptor. She embodies in herself everything she offers others. Her authority, her authenticity, her personal commitment and presence entrain just about everyone into the beauty already to be found in their lives, often obscured, however, by the shadow of disease and the ghosts of fear, pain, and turmoil accompanying it. She titled her previous book *Here for Now*. That says it all.

Seven years later, Elana is still here for now, very much alive, indeed brimming with life and with a hard-earned wisdom and kindness. Here, in these pages, she shares with you the essence of what she has learned from being well even when she was sick, and from being well now, even with the perpetual uncertainly of future test results. The text is made even sweeter and richer through the stories of her interactions with her patients and with the participants in her MBSR classes, when her voice and theirs, and her heart and theirs, seem to join in poignant recognitions, realizations, and reconcilings.

This is a subtle and powerful book, a masterpiece of simplicity, clarity, and caring that only Elana could have authored, being who she is, and given everything she has had to face and work with over the years. It is profoundly inspiring and at the same time, extremely practical. The real secret of her work, as you will soon learn, is that what she is teaching can and needs to be cultivated. Mindfulness is not merely a good idea. It is a way of being, as in "well-being" and in "being well." Here is Elana to guide you in its cultivation and in befriending what is deepest and best and most healing in yourself.

Jon Kabat-Zinn
Berkeley, California
February 2012

Acknowledgments

I am blessed to be among many people who have helped this book come into being. My parents, now deceased, led the way, leaving me a legacy of love and generosity. Their lifetime of caring and compassion taught me to trust the innate goodness of people and maintain an open heart. My husband, David, has been a constant source of comfort and joy. He has sat by my bed and stood by my side with a steadiness of care and devotion that enriches my life and supports all that I do. I am grateful to my brother Bob, a truly wise and loving brother, whose wisdom and counsel has been invaluable. I thank him for his input and suggestions. I feel very fortunate that we share the same path.

I'd like to thank all my patients who have entrusted me with their care and let me enter into their world so honestly and directly. Their stories are woven throughout this book as sources of inspiration and examples of courage and perseverance. In particular I'd like to thank Laura McNaughton, MaryAnn Pendleton, Pam Spielberg, and Cindy Taberner. I honor the memory of Stephanie Stuhr Colson, who maintained light and love until the very end. She is missed, as is Suzanne Patton, whose clarity and care for family never abated. Ann Fernbach, my cousin, added her eloquence and honesty by sharing her thoughts to me as she underwent treatment for cancer. Diane Reibel and Margaret Cullen, fellow meditators, teachers, and cancer survivors, were generous in sharing their experience and knowledge.

My stem-cell sisters, Peggy Steinberger, Janet Birbara, Agneta Brown, and Linda Pape, all contributed to this book and continue to add support, richness, and great dinners to my life. The Berklee wonder women—Sheila Katz, Suzanne Hanser, Sally Blazer, and Rebecca Perricone—cheered me on through all the stages of writing.

I am honored to know a group of dedicated hospice social workers—Caryn Stewart, Suzanne Doiron-Schiavone, Elizabeth Rotti, Lynn Mazur, and Nicole Karaku—who have taught me much about the challenges of illness and being present to help a person die with dignity and care. I also thank the Worcester VNA nurses, social workers, and staff, who are dedicating themselves to their patients and teaching me about compassionate care.

I appreciate and applaud all the men and women who have attended classes through the many years in the Stress Reduction Program at the University of Massachusetts Center for Mindfulness. You have been my teachers, proving to me that suffering is optional and mindfulness transformative no matter what the problem.

This book and the thoughts and practices contained within would not be here without the influence of Jon Kabat-Zinn. I thank him for being my friend and teacher all these years. His wisdom, generosity, and leadership in bringing mindfulness into the world sets an example for myself and others to follow. I also bow to Saki Santorelli, director of the Center for Mindfulness and my longtime friend and colleague, for extending the reach of the center and helping so many thrive through its programs.

I feel lucky to be a part of a community of MBSR teachers who share the goal of relieving suffering. I have spent many hours discussing how best to accomplish this with my dear friends and fellow teachers, Florence Meleo-Meyer, Zayda Vallejo, Melissa Blacker, and

Diana Kamila, as well as Ferris Buck Urbanoski and all the other teachers here in Worcester and the far reaches of the world. The world of psychotherapy also informs my work. My friends Susan Rashba and Chris Nevins Bright are gifted therapists and very caring friends. Thank you for your insight and support over the years.

Susan Bauer Wu has allowed my experience on the bone marrow transplant unit to be translated into a study bringing mindfulness to patients undergoing a stem cell transplant. Her friendship and shared mission extends the reach and understanding of mindfulness and adds joy to the process.

My oncologist, Arnie Freedman, helps my body stay well and is also receptive to the heart and mind of healing. I appreciate his openness and willingness to listen, care, and explore new ideas.

I'd like to thank Eden Steinberg, who approached me with the idea for this book and ushered it into Shambhala for publication; Beth Frankl, my editor, who brought it to fruition; and assistant editor Ben Gleason. My agent, Stephanie Tade, has given me wise counsel and supported my efforts. Laurie Porter, a good friend, was invaluable in helping me with my first draft and encouraging my effort. Naomi Litrownik taught me about commas and gave me a book on grammar.

It is impossible to do this work alone, and there are many who have supported this work. Please forgive me for not mentioning your name. Your gifts of love, thought, and action are held in my heart. I am forever grateful.

Being Well (Even When You're Sick)

Introduction

Mindfulness has helped me have a life—and I mean this literally. I have lived with non-Hodgkin's lymphoma since 1995, and without the ability to quiet my mind and cope with the stress of illness, I truly don't believe I would be here. My first book, *Here for Now: Living Well with Cancer through Mindfulness,* is about how I applied the mindfulness-based stress reduction (MBSR) program in coping with all the ups and downs of cancer through my initial diagnosis, a stem cell transplant, recovery, and adjustment to a new normal.

This book includes the work I've done with people in my practice of mindfulness-based psychotherapy and stress reduction. It's challenging to live with a serious disease and want to maintain a state of well-being. Every day I am aware that I can have a recurrence at any moment; I will be sick again and may die sooner than I wish. This has motivated me to write this book and convey what I have learned personally and from others. Every moment is meaningful. As you read along and practice the meditations, know that you are not alone. There is a community of people practicing along with you and wishing you well.

This book is not a manual. There are no quick fixes or miracle techniques to being mindful. My intention is to inspire hope and to help you feel in charge of your life and connect to your innate wisdom and joy. I encourage you to pause, breathe, and appreciate your own being and your willingness for self-exploration. Every breath offers opportunities for a new perspective that is life enhancing. Meditation is an invaluable part of this process. I encourage you to do the meditations I have recorded for this book (available for download at www.shambhala.com/BeingWell) regularly so they can become part of your day. Forms of these meditations have been used for thousands of years. But their presentation here comes from my heart-mind and my experience working with my own unruly self to cultivate patience, compassion, and acceptance. May your life be enriched through them as have mine and others who believe they are well even when they're sick. Thank you for sharing this journey with me. May we all be well.

1 / Mindfulness

Mindfulness represents not only mind but also the totality of our experience in relating to the world through all the senses. It is not a static "thing" to obtain but rather a lively and dynamic process of living fully. By being mindful, we are choosing to be awake and connected, connected to the workings of the mind and body as well as to the nature of things as they are. Jon Kabat-Zinn, my dear friend and colleague, defines mindfulness as "a conscious bringing of attention to the present moment without judgment." This requires a fierce but loving attention to *all* that arises in mind and body, whether we like it or not. The more we resist what we don't like and try to change the unchangeable, the more we tense up and create suffering.

Understanding and compassion in noticing *all the mind states* that arise as moments unfold one by one is part of being mindful. Such compassion is essential, because some of what arises is inevitably difficult to accept. Mindfulness has to be practical, showing how it is beneficial to be able to continually pay attention and open to the reality of our lives. To notice what is here now, in this moment, is to open to the pleasant and the unpleasant, the good and the bad. I think of it as a dance. We are always coordinating our steps to the rhythm of life, trying to keep the beat and stay in step with the changing tempo. When we flow with it, there is harmony. Mindfulness creates harmony and brings joy—if we also allow ourselves to experience sadness.

When I am talking about being mindful, I always tell the story,

"Good, Bad, Who Knows?" Since 1984, I have taught at the Center for Mindfulness's Stress Reduction Clinic in Worcester, Massachusetts. Often I meet people who have been in one of my classes. Whether it is on the street or in the supermarket, they invariably stop to say hello and tell me, "I still return to my breath when I'm upset, and I remember the story you told us about the farmer whose horse ran away."

As many times as I have told this story, it remains relevant. When the farmer's friends came to express pity for his bad luck, he said, "Good, bad, who knows?" When the horse returned and brought with it a herd of horses, people came to congratulate him on his good luck. Again, he said, "Good, bad, who knows?" Some time later, one of the new horses kicked his son and broke his leg. As people expressed sympathy, the farmer said, "Good, bad, who knows?" Good things happened, bad things happened, and his response never changed. At the end of the story, all the boys of the village were conscripted and sent to war except the farmer's son. "Good, bad, who knows?"

I smile when I hear that this story continues to have resonance for my former students. It raises such important questions. How can we ever consider something bad, like cancer, good? Is it possible to maintain equanimity in the face of bad news? How do we deal with loss, disappointment, and possibly death and maintain calm? Is it possible? Does this mindfulness thing really help? After all, it doesn't change anything.

Mindfulness is not about an absence of emotion or a way to stem the natural flow of illness, aging, loss, and separation. This flow may be inevitable, but our response to it is not. I live this truth. I take it to heart. As a person who lives with cancer and the uncertainty of another recurrence, I need to be mindful. This "bad" thing (cancer) is also "good," because it forces me to remember that my time is limited. Knowing this is a gift that forces me to notice what brings joy and harmony and what does not. This is mindfulness: learning from what we do and acknowledging the patterns of thought and action that have been established so we can decide whether they continue to serve us well.

Many people think that the mind must remain blank and quiet to engage successfully in the practice of mindfulness. This is only a thought—or perhaps a wish—and can cause striving and false expectations that, in turn, create suffering. It is normal for the mind to wander. In fact, during meditation and mindfulness practice, the mind is sometimes referred to as "monkey mind," because it naturally moves all over the place, jumping from one thought or feeling to another. This is not a problem unless we think it should not happen. With patience and acceptance, the mind does begin to quiet, but not if we try to push it away or repress it. If we try to control it, it will, like a rebellious child, refuse to calm. Trying to force a thought away rather than noting it and observing its effect on the body is harsh and self-defeating; moreover, it stops us from learning about the pattern of our thinking. It is more useful to acknowledge thought and escort our attention back to the breath or a more neutral object of attention in our immediate experience. We can also name the thought, calling it worry, judgment, plan, memory, fear, or expectation. Or we can quietly say, "Thinking" or "Habit," and investigate how the mind's activity is affecting our body.

I remember leaving every morning for a job I didn't like and thinking, "I wish I didn't have to go to work." Once I noticed this pattern, I could instead concentrate on entering the car, starting it up, feeling the seat underneath me and my hands on the steering wheel, looking out at the road ahead. I passed some beautiful scenery on the road to work, but I hadn't even noticed it. Eventually, I changed jobs, but before that was possible, I needed to change my view, both literally and figuratively. When we are ill, it is even more important to observe our thoughts rather than being drawn into them and mistaking thought for reality. How often we focus on what could go wrong or a loss we have had instead of focusing on the fact that we are *here*. The ability to stop, pause, and take a breath is calming. I get anxious days before I have a CT scan. I must consciously stop and remind myself not to jump ahead. I may not know what the test will show, but I can feel my breath, taste my food, and smile at my husband. He likes this approach too. If I stay calm, he is also better able to manage his concern that I will be ill again.

Mindfulness is not merely a technique or only about relaxation. As we tell people who are entering the mindfulness-based stress reduction (MBSR) program, "Do not try too hard to relax; this will only cause tension." It seems counterintuitive to allow yourself to be on edge or notice a negative thought or feeling without trying to change it. But forcing yourself to relax when you feel nervous is like having a gun pointed at your head and being told, "Don't worry."

It is true that a calm, clear, and more serene mind is an outcome of mindfulness meditation, but the ultimate goal of this practice is heightened awareness to feel more alive and be free of suffering. It is a practice that cultivates compassion and wisdom.

Mindfulness is an adventure.

The present moment is a precious moment.

Let's begin.

Awareness Exercise

Where are you right now? When you look around, what do you see? Can you hear any sounds, and if so, are they constant or do they change?

What is the position of your body? Are there any parts of your body that you feel more than others? Can you bring attention to any sensations that are present? Do they change? Are you responding in any particular way to these sensations? Do you wish they would change? Do you find them pleasant, unpleasant, or neutral?

Are you having any thoughts? If you were to label them, what would you call them? Do they have a temporal quality (are they in the past or the future)? What are their qualities? Are they effecting any changes in your body?

Can you feel yourself breathing? What are you noticing about your breath? What is its rhythm? Is it long or short, even or choppy? How long is the inhalation? The exhalation? What are its qualities? Can you feel the pause between the breaths?

Are you interested? Can you be curious? Are you willing not to know what will happen next? Can you be free of judging, and if not, can you accept and not judge the judging?

Pause, listen, look, allow, and trust what emerges. You can be free of suffering.

2 / Taking Control

Setting Goals and Intentions

Who is rich?
He who rejoices in his portion.

—*Talmudic saying*

He who controls others may be powerful, but he who has mastered himself is mightier still.

—*Lao Tzu*

Bringing mindfulness into a hospital setting was radical back in 1979, when Jon Kabat-Zinn combined his knowledge of microbiology and meditation into a new program he called mindfulness-based stress reduction at the University of Massachusetts Medical School. Working as a scientist at the school, he observed the suffering of the patients who came for help, as well as the reactions of the doctors, nurses, and other professionals who cared for them. Jon brought with him not only scientific training but also a strong practice of mindfulness. This practice, which is more than two thousand years old, can be long and complex with many rituals and belief systems, but it is also very simple—be here now, fully and wholly. Jon saw the effect of meditation in his life and those of his friends and felt that difficulties could be met and suffering minimized with a willingness to be daring and face the circumstances of our lives with acceptance and mindfulness.

This belief led him to redirect attention to the mind-body connection by creating a program that would empower patients to take more responsibility for their own healing and complement medical interventions. He secured the support of hospital administration and MBSR began in 1979. This program is now established throughout the world and has been researched and proven effective in easing the suffering of many disorders, both psychological and medical.

The first patients who came to the program did so because their doctors despaired of helping them. They had chronic pain or other disease-related symptoms that were not amenable to treatment. At the time, I was working as a psychotherapist in a large HMO down the road from the medical school. I was struggling with my own frustration at the lack of communication between doctors, who focused on the physical, and we psychotherapists, who concentrated on mental health. The emphasis was on fixing what was wrong rather than focusing on what was right. I discovered that MBSR did the opposite. It integrated the mind and the body and built on a person's strengths, assuming that everyone was already whole and had what they needed to be well. This was within each person's control and ability.

I listened to my heart and head and quit my therapy job at the HMO and, in 1984, began teaching with Jon and Saki Santorelli at the Stress Reduction Clinic. When I began teaching, I had no idea that mindfulness would infiltrate my own belief system and permeate every pore of my being. I only knew that it always kept me challenged and engaged. I loved teaching and investigating what helped a person, me included, be well. This outlook and experience served me well when I became a patient myself and had a chance to test its efficacy. I never chose to have cancer, but when I was diagnosed in 1995 with non-Hodgkin's lymphoma, I knew that I could take control of my own well-being by being mindful and living what I taught. I consciously chose to live as fully as possible, even with cancer and the uncertainty of my longevity. My motto became "Yes to life and all that's in it."

Author Isaac Bashevis Singer was once asked, "Do you believe in free will?" He responded, "Sure I do, it's the only choice I have."

I love this quote. It reminds me that we all have choices, but as much as we plan and do our best to control events, the unexpected happens, such as learning we have a life-threatening illness. What we took for granted is no longer certain, but we can choose how we relate to it.

One evening, a patient of mine who worried about dying because she had metastatic breast cancer was driving home after visiting her mother. The visit had gone well, and she was feeling content and peaceful when a deer struck her windshield. Her car was totaled, but miraculously, she was unhurt. As she examined the dead deer at the side of the road, she was filled with gratitude at being spared. Suddenly, cancer became less of a threat, and she gained a new perspective and greater appreciation of her life. She gave the deer to a traveler who stopped to help her and was ecstatic to live for another day.

Control is a myth, and yet it is real. Having a sense of control is like riding a bike over varied terrain—it changes and we change. To remain balanced, we're constantly adjusting our position, shifting gears, and altering our pace and speed. This takes practice, but the more we ride, the more skillful and confident we become.

There is much research being done now on resilience, which is what helps us cope with difficult times. One of the early researchers in this field is Susan Kobasa, a professor at the City University of

New York. She felt it would be useful to study people who successfully navigated difficult times, and in the late 1970s, she carried out
a study on a group of executives who were under a lot of stress while
their company underwent radical restructuring. On completion of
the study, she found that certain personality traits protected some of
the executives and managers from the health ravages of stress. She
termed these characteristics "stress hardiness," and they included the
following:

1. Commitment
2. Control
3. Challenge

Learning to control how we react to the challenges we face in a
more flexible, more confident, and less destructive way leads to stress
hardiness. Our intention to do what we can to be well and maintain a
state of well-being is under our control. Doing so is challenging, and we
need to be willing to meet what arises. If you're reading this book, the
likelihood is that either you or someone you love is sick, has been sick,
or fears being sick. Our goal is to navigate the road of illness to well-
being skillfully. Intention can fuel our journey, pointing us in the right
direction and helping us persevere even when we feel like quitting.

The following are intentions that I have found helpful. I recommend reading through them, evaluating what is meaningful to you,
and observing what resonates. You are invited to use them as guides.
If you like, you can jot down your own intentions to use as signposts
to keep you headed in the right direction. Even if you have doubts
as to their achievability, write them down. You may be surprised at
the results.

MY INTENTIONS

1. I will be responsible for my own well-being and act to free myself from suffering. I will commit to doing what is possible to meet the truth of the moment with acceptance and compassion.

2. I will persevere and not give up, especially when I am feeling hopeless and discouraged, angry, frustrated, or hurt. The new moment is a fresh opportunity to pick myself up and try again. I will be open to new perspectives and, like the GPS in my car, recalculate.

3. I will acknowledge expectations, wishes, and shoulds. I will feel whatever emotions arise and observe them with the intention of learning from them and my conditioned patterns of response. I will be open to, allow, and observe what is negative as well as positive.

4. I will cultivate affectionate attention. I will be kind to myself, caring and compassionate. I will treat myself as if I were comforting someone dear and beloved, like cradling an infant in my arms, holding her close and learning what soothes this being who is hurting and afraid. I will be forgiving and compassionate to pain that is self-inflicted or caused by the ignorance and fears of others. I will soften, allow, and treasure this sensitive, vulnerable part of myself, being supported and supportive of what arises. It will pass.

5. I will reside in the present moment as if it were my home and practice coming home with patience and diligence. I will cultivate calm and attention and sustain it by focusing on a single object such as my breath. My breath will become an anchor to keep me steady regardless of circumstances.

6. I will practice remembering that everything changes, but I am here now. Peace lies within this moment. I will have faith in my own wisdom, strength, and ability to know what is wholesome and healthy.

7. I will remember that I can't control events but I can choose how I relate to them.

What are your intentions? I recommend taking some moments to sit quietly, giving your intentions permission to emerge freely. You can write them down and revisit or alter them as often as you like.

My intention is:

- Be kind to myself
- to live in the moment & not look too far ahead
- Be less negative about the future and my physical issues
- feeling change is positive if painful.

My intention is:

_____

_____

_____

_____

_____

My intention is:

_____

_____

_____

_____

_____

_____

I recommend posting these intentions in a place that is visible, where they can inspire and guide you in being well.

3 / Commitment

The moment one definitely commits oneself, then Providence moves too. All sorts of things occur to help one that would never otherwise have occurred. A whole stream of events issues from the decision, raising in one's favor all manner of unforeseen incidents and meetings and material assistance, which no one could have dreamed would have come their way.
—*Johann Wolfgang von Goethe*

He'd fly through the air with the greatest of ease,
That daring young man on the flying trapeze.
—*Popular song of the nineteenth century*

News like a diagnosis of cancer can make you feel suspended between the life you have known and the life that will be. It can seem as though everything is up in the air, making it difficult to make plans or decide on treatment options. The thought of moving through this experience with ease may seem improbable, yet it is possible. It does, however, take daring to move through worry and fear and master it. When you are in the midst of negative thoughts and feelings, it is difficult to have faith that it will pass. Making that leap takes courage—and practice. Each time you catch yourself flying into the arms of fear and are willing to examine it, respect its power, *and breathe with it,* you are letting it move around you like molecules of air. Ease comes by relaxing into, rather than away from, difficulty. STOP is an acronym you will see throughout this book. When you see it, stop, take a breath, open to and observe your experience, and then proceed. Committing yourself to this practice will help you recenter yourself with ease.

· · · · · · · · · · ·

Stop.
Take a breath.
Open and observe.
Proceed.

Can you feel your breath now?
What thoughts are present as you read this?
Do you dare to notice what arises as it is arising—like now?
Are you willing to commit yourself to this process and take that leap?

· · · · · · · · · · ·

Sherry came to the Stress Reduction Clinic to learn MBSR after seeing numerous doctors and experiencing many failed attempts to get relief from pain. For her, physical suffering was compounded by a sense of futility and loss. A few years before, after many years of being single, she had met a man she loved and married. He was much older than she, and within a year, he died. His grown children had never liked her and resented the marriage. Now they were fighting with her over his estate. She also was in litigation over a recent car accident that had left her with residual injuries. Angry and bitter, Sherry seemed to focus most of her energy on these battles and how awful her life was. When she entered my office and sat down, she told me that she didn't think MBSR could help her, but her doctor had tried everything else and nothing had worked.

She reported that this was the first time she had left her house in a long time. She had stopped working and couldn't even see friends because of severe pain in her back and neck. It had effectively halted her life as she had known it. She felt alone and powerless. She was involved in a legal battle that was stressful. Home alone, her mind focused on the unfairness of life and the misery of her circumstances. I asked her if she had sought psychiatric help. She said she hadn't; her primary care physician had prescribed some medication for depression, but it hadn't helped. She didn't believe psychotherapy—or anything else—could help her. All her attention was focused on her physical pain.

At the Stress Reduction Clinic, we ask participants to commit to an eight-week program. There are twenty-eight hours of class time, which include one all-day session and forty-five minutes of daily homework. Each class focuses on an essential element of mindfulness and provides experiences and discussions. The emphasis is on self-responsibility and accountability.

Core beliefs are as follows:

1. There is more right with us than wrong.
2. We are not our disease.
3. We have the power to effect change.
4. We are responsible for our actions and the consequences of our actions.

As I sat with Sherry, explaining this approach and describing the use of breath and the cultivation of attention and acceptance, I felt her doubt and a heaviness—not just of extra pounds but also of negativity, helplessness, and anger. The mental and physical were intertwined; it would take effort for her to enter into these feelings without fleeing from them or judging herself harshly.

"Do you really want to do this?" I asked her. "It requires discipline and effort. It is not easy. You'll have to promise to use the CD we give you and do the different meditations, awareness of breathing, a mental scan of your body, some yoga or walking meditations, and daily awareness exercises."

Misery and her doctor's recommendation prompted her to say, "Yes, MBSR is my last resort."

I explained that she would have to take time for herself *every day* to do nothing but quietly observe what arose and allow herself to experience it as well as her reactions. Her thoughts and sensations would include feelings, some pleasant, some unpleasant. She would be witnessing them and letting them move on, flowing through her mind and body.

"This takes practice," I said, "and patience. You can turn the CD off at any time, but minds can be like monkeys, going all over the place unexpectedly. Can you be curious about this mind as if it were a new acquaintance? Are you open to making friends with it and learning more about its patterns of thought?"

For Sherry, "yes" meant a commitment to caring for herself, to giving mindfulness a chance. "Yes" was the beginning of change, interrupting the cycle of paralysis and negativity that was perpetuating her suffering. "Yes" meant acknowledging that she did have some control;

she didn't need to remain stuck in the past; instead, there were possibilities now in her present.

Sherry said, "Yes." She came to class regularly and used the guided meditations. One day she came in smiling, her energy level clearly much higher. She proudly reported, "I realize I am not my pain. I still have pain, but it isn't me."

Since that time, Sherry has reengaged in life. She still lives alone, but now she goes out with friends and is busy with different activities. She eventually lost her court case, but by then she had decided it no longer affected her happiness. She continues to meditate and refreshes her practice by playing her CD or returning to the Stress Reduction Clinic for an all-day session or graduate class. Most important, her attitude has shifted. She still experiences pain, yet she is well and living a full life—with pain. She now knows that she is more than her pain.

You do not need to take the eight-week program to know that it is possible to take control of your life and differentiate your disease and its symptoms from the totality of your being. I have adapted MBSR as I sit with patients on a one-to-one basis in my office, in the hospital, or in their home. You can do it yourself by reading this book and following the meditations available for download at www.shambhala .com/BeingWell—if you make the commitment to do so. It's your choice and within your control. What do you believe? Remember your intentions and goals. What is your commitment to yourself?

Can you believe the thought of "I am more than my pain, my cancer, my dis-ease?" Can you believe that it is possible to be well, even now? Are you willing to explore mindfulness to help you live with ease?

If the answer is "yes," I recommend taking out your journal and writing down your commitment to yourself. Write as quickly as you can without censoring what comes up. Put it aside and then do it again every day this week. If it is too hard for you to write or it is not your way, mentally make a commitment to yourself that you can repeat each day. You may repeat it as often as you like. You can write your commitment on stickers and place them in strategic locations as a reminder. Choose a word or phrase that can be repeated in times of difficulty, or simply hold and cherish it with appreciation for your willingness to engage in this process of being well.

Reflection: What Does It Mean to Be Well?

Take a moment and allow yourself to be aware of your breathing; without trying to change anything, let your mind settle into this moment. You can begin by noting the flow of breath and where you feel it most vividly in the body. As your attention rests with the breath, let yourself experience the inhalation, noting the air as it enters the body and its path as it leaves the body, observing the length, the pace, and the pause before it becomes an exhalation. Feel the rhythm of your breath, allowing it to flow naturally and without effort, experiencing the sense of being breathed. When you notice your awareness has moved away, gently but firmly return to the experience of breathing. You can notice where the breath is most vivid for you and observe its effect on the body, noticing how and where it moves the body. Let thoughts come and go, noting them but continuing to use your breath as your central focus of attention. Let yourself open to whatever enters your awareness, letting your breath anchor you to the moment so you can more readily observe the sea of change.

If you like, you can note how many breaths you feel before a thought enters your awareness. Can you stop the thought from happening? What happens if you try? What sensations are present? If you are experiencing a strong sensation, you can gently breathe with it, opening and allowing it rather than trying to change it. When you're ready, let the breath again be your center of attention. Does this take effort? Do you find this process interesting or not? Notice how your attitude toward this exercise affects the way you feel.

Once you have reached a level of attention where you feel quiet and calm, ask yourself, "What does it mean to be well?"

VISUALIZING AND SENSING WELLNESS NOTE

What sensations are present?

How do you look?

What are you doing?

Are you alone or with others?

What is the environment around you?

What feeling are present?

What emotions can you name as you experience this sense of health?

What thoughts are present?

How much of wellness is dependent on physical health?

Is there sadness, resignation, or disappointment because your picture of yourself well is not congruent with the way you are right now?

What is the time frame? Is it a time in the past or the future? Can you feel it now?

Return to your breath and allow your attention to rest here, noting what arises. Continue to allow the breath to be your primary focus of attention and remember to have it rest here in the present moment for a few minutes, noticing what is present. When you're ready, open your eyes if they are closed. You may then do the following writing exercise.

Writing Exercise

When you are ready, take out your pen and paper and write down what arose as you asked yourself what it means to be well. Write quickly and spontaneously for three minutes. When you are done, pause, review what you wrote, and pause again. Then ask yourself, "How can I maintain this sense of well-being?" Write for another three minutes and then put the paper aside. This exercise can be repeated at another time.

Making a commitment to being well and forming this intention from an inner place of knowing is powerful. It is a beacon to follow in times of hardship and sorrow, when we lose faith as well as when we feel joyous and strong.

4 / Making Practice Practical

If you have built castles in the air, your work need not be lost; that is where they should be. Now put the foundations under them.

You must live in the present, launch yourself on every wave, find your eternity in each moment.

—*Henry David Thoreau*

My patients laugh at me because, every now and then, they catch me taking a deep breath and slowly exhaling. I admit that I may exaggerate the out-breath somewhat, but I do it to signal to a patient that we're on a runaway train and it's time to stop and reflect. I turn to my breath because my body is giving me a message. It could be a heaviness in the middle of my chest, a tension in my shoulders, or a tightness in my belly. As a patient describes a fight with a spouse or trouble with a child, I notice I am reliving the problem along with him. I react to what I am hearing physically and so intensely that my ability to be a reflecting mirror is lost. My cue to stop and take a breath is the contraction in my belly or observing that my shoulders are at my ears, my body leaning forward, and my heart beating more rapidly. The moment I become aware of these physical signals, I stop. As I exhale, I am releasing tension and recentering myself. And as I stop and calm, so can my patients. Then we can problem solve.

Mindfulness is practical. It comes in handy as we undergo procedures, wait in doctors' offices, or deal with family and friends who may be even more distraught about our illness than we are. Personally, it helps me know that a problem is solvable and that my fearful, anxious state will pass.

When I sit with patients, teaching them about mindfulness, I never really explain it in words. Instead, with their permission, we meet each other eye to eye and heart to heart, and I demonstrate the practice. My task is to help them connect to what they need and help them experience this moment—the present moment—as a home where they can relax and renew. No one wants to suffer unnecessarily. I too have been subjected to tests, long periods of waiting for doctors or test results, and the effects of chemotherapy. I know how hard it is to maintain perspective and be a patient. Wellness can seem like a dream—Walt Disney's creation of Cinderella's castle, beautiful but imaginary. Our task in being mindful is to create a foundation that is stable and calm, so our dream is a reality experienced every day and throughout the day, moment by moment.

Knowledge is key. So is practice.

Sickness affects the mind and body so that our mental acuity and sense of control and optimism can be dulled or depressed along with bodily ills. We are vulnerable. In a strange new land with many unknowns, the self we've known is changed, and we may often be dependent on others to assist us in living. This sense of helplessness can intensify symptoms and the emotions that accompany them. Much of how we relate to the conditions of our illness depends on past learning. Often unconsciously, we tend to retreat into our default position, whatever that may be for each of us. Mine was to push ahead as if my strength hadn't changed. I needed friends to remind me that it was OK to rest and my mindfulness practice to remind me to truly listen to my body and respond accordingly.

Mindfulness, practiced regularly, wakes us up to our automatic pilot. The body is the red light telling us to stop, pay attention, and pause before we repeat behaviors that are no longer useful. It is our friend, cuing us to our emotions so we have more mastery over them.

I explain to patients that noticing their own attitudes, beliefs, and ways of processing information can be helpful to them. "Mindfulness is a way of paying attention on purpose to the present moment without being judgmental and with acceptance," I say. "What are you aware of right now?"

Often, the answer is an emotional one, mental rather than tangible or observable. I may then redirect their attention to a specific element in the room, perhaps a sound. I ask patients to listen to what their ears are receiving. If we are in the hospital, it might be the clicking of machines or nurses talking nearby, whatever is occurring at the time.

Sound is a good place to start in understanding what it means to be mindful. It is outside ourselves and happens on its own without our needing to do anything except be willing to listen. This evokes a receptive attitude that is free of striving. The intention to listen is enough. Sound comes to you.

"What do you notice now as you look around?" I ask after we've explored the sounds in the room. Then, depending on time and response, we might move on to breath and then to sensations.

The place is the present and the object explored is what is currently immediate and available. Sometimes, if I sense there is high anxiety, I will help a person calm by putting her hand on her belly and feeling what happens as she breathes in and out. My voice is steady and calm and matches the slowing of the breath as we go along breath by breath. I want people to listen to their own internal cues to return to this moment and this breath as the anchor to the present moment. It's practical to stay with our breathing because it's here, right now. It changes, we change, and yet it goes on as long as we are alive. The more we can experience it and use it to fix our attention, the more it benefits us in times of need. It is a reminder: I'm here!

If a patient expresses a strong emotion, I acknowledge it. I know it will pass, but I hope that he will realize this as well. Rather than delve into the whys and whats of the feeling, which only prolongs it, I help him know that he can examine the feeling as it is expressed in the body and shift attention to its physical manifestation.

"What sensations are present?" I ask.

This question shifts attention from the mind to the body. It puts some distance between thought and feeling, which makes it more manageable. (I shall discuss this more later. It's a way to work with strong emotion.) We accept whatever is being felt. We can learn from it and know that it is transitory. There is no wrong response. Everything that occurs is an opportunity for mindfulness.

Let's pause for a moment now and let this information settle.

. . . .

STOP, TAKE A BREATH, OPEN AND OBSERVE, AND PROCEED

As you stop, take a breath and tune in to your experience. What are you observing? Where is your awareness? Are you hearing sounds? Are you experiencing any sensations, and, if so, where are they located? How would you describe the sensation? What is its duration and intensity?

Are you aware of thinking? Is it a single thought or a stream of thoughts? Does it have an emotional component? If so, can you feel it physically and locate it in your body? Is there any constriction or tightness? Simply note what occurs and continue doing so for at least a minute. What are you observing now? Can you accept it?

Let's pause again. Can you feel your breath? How long can you follow it before a thought pops in? Can you do this without judging yourself, allowing it to be as it is and yourself to be as you are, or are you trying to make something happen? Simply observe; you are practicing mindfulness.

Remember, you can pause any time you want or need to regain composure. As you pause, you don't have to feel breath; instead, you can be aware of sound, locate an object of attention or even find your feet, look at an object in the room, gaze at the sky, or meet a loved one's eyes. You get to choose what it is that refocuses your attention on the here and now. This is grounding and helps expand your perspective. Pausing gives you this moment—and the next— to take that breath, open and observe, and then proceed with greater calm. Simple is good. Mindfulness need not be complicated. The less you struggle, the more energy you have available for healing.

When you are very sick, concentration is fleeting, but it is still possible to be mindful. Mindfulness may mean listening to the clicking of a machine or looking at a calming object either in or outside of the room. Having a person next to you who is quietly sitting and caring can make a difference. This silent presence is also mindfulness.

. . . .

Recently I had the privilege of being the consultant to a large study that investigated the use of mindfulness to alleviate the considerable emotional and physical pain of people who are undergoing a stem cell transplant experience. This is an inpatient procedure of intensive chemotherapy lasting anywhere from three to five weeks. Cancer cells are destroyed, but so is the immune system. Immunity is then rebuilt by reinserting the patient's own cells (stem cells that regenerate), which were extracted from the patient prior to the procedure. In working with these patients and teaching them mindfulness, we were well aware of how ill they were. Sometimes we would just sit quietly with them, encouraging them to breathe with their pain and not struggle unnecessarily. Patients were often reluctant to have a witness to their suffering. It is unpleasant to be nauseous or have chills or burning sensations, but agitation makes it worse. Discovering that calm is possible is very useful, but in the beginning, this can be a leap of faith. Breathing with and softening into pain can be threatening. It is helpful to have a coach. Knowing when to accept help is part of being mindful. Acceptance is neither automatic nor easy, but the more we understand what helps us be calm instead of beating up on ourselves when we fail, the easier it will be to tolerate our illness. It helps to remember to STOP and bring attention to when we feel good as well as bad. The greater our repertoire of responses, the more control we have in maintaining perspective and calm.

A patient who was in our feasibility study told the interviewer, "Sometimes I'd listen to the breath of the air and the wind blowing, and the calmness of the whole thing just put me in a different mindset, and I found that very relaxing."

. . . .

In-breath, out-breath,
I can stop and refocus my attention.
In-breath, out-breath,

I need not struggle.
In-breath, out-breath,
I am worthy
of love and peace.
In-breath, out-breath,
I am here.
I am well.

· · · · · · · · · ·

Awareness Practice

To cultivate this ability to pay attention with an attitude of curiosity, wonder, and acceptance, it is useful to practice on something outside ourselves that is familiar and doesn't arouse strong feelings. In the first MBSR class of each session at the Stress Reduction Clinic, we use a raisin, an object that all of us have experienced and that can be explored with all of our five senses. Participants are given three raisins and asked to imagine that, like a small child or a being from another planet, they have never seen or felt these objects before and are being exposed to them for the first time. Their task is to discover whether a raisin is harmful by exploring it carefully:

Look at the object, noting its color(s) and shape.
Feel it, exploring its texture, firmness and softness, ridges and valleys.
Smell it.
Listen to see if it makes a sound.

Notice all you can about it, and if you like, jot down what you observe. You can hold the object to your ear to see if it makes a sound, manipulate it, smell it, and see if all of the objects are the same. (Do not put it in your mouth until instructed to do so.)

Now identify one of the objects to place in your mouth.
Note the choosing of the object.
Bring attention to picking it up and placing it in your hand.
Note as you aim it toward your mouth and place it in your mouth.
Let it rest on your tongue.

Can you note what it is like and experience having it in your mouth *before* you bite into it? What does it feel like? Does it have a taste? Where is the taste located on your tongue? Do you notice anything else? Are there any associations?

Take one bite; pause; and note the new experience created by this action, how the object has changed, how the perception of it changes as your awareness does.
Continue exploring the process of biting, chewing, and swallowing until the object is no longer in your mouth.
Repeat this process with the two remaining objects.

What have you observed? What have you learned?
I offer people the opportunity to do this exercise three times: the first slowly while following my instructions, the second slowly on their own, and the third any way they want. Usually, people discover that their "normal" way of eating is too fast and that they don't have as intense or vivid an experience as when they mindfully and slowly are present with each step of the process of holding, choosing, and ingesting the object.

"What did you notice?" I ask them.

"It has more than one color."

"It's dry. Are these old?"

"You should use organic raisins!"

"I usually gulp these down and never taste them."

"I eat too fast."

"The first bite was a taste explosion."

"I never liked raisins, but this didn't taste the way I expected it to."

Some people love raisins; some hate them. Some refuse to do the exercise, while others do it and are angry they are asked to do it.

I acknowledge each comment.

"How interesting," I say.

Often, people are astonished to discover the uniqueness of each raisin and the variability of their experience as they choose one, place it in their mouth, and ingest it.

I have done this awareness exercise hundreds of times in many different settings—in the medical school, in the stress reduction program, in hospitals with patients, and in workshops attended by health care professionals. It is always interesting and always a learning experience for the person doing it as well as for me. The object need not be a raisin. When I do this exercise with people on the bone marrow transplant unit, I use an ice chip. They wouldn't be able to chew a raisin; their mouths are too covered with sores. So we use what is soothing and available. All patients have a cup filled with ice chips on the tray in their room, and we ask that they lift the cup, look inside, and explore the ice chips. They then get to choose one, pick it up, notice how it is placed either in a spoon or in their hand, and examine it with their eyes and fingers. Observing the ice with all their senses, they can even bring it up to their ear and listen for any sound that might be present. Patients observe how it changes and, when they're ready, choose a chip and consciously transfer it to their mouth. Closing their eyes, they continue attending to its process of transformation. We then discuss it, and I invite them to do this on their own. The purpose of this exercise is to see the familiar with fresh eyes and a new perspective that we hope can generalize to the challenge of illness.

· · · · · · · · · · ·

SENSORY AWARENESS

Choose a familiar object that you can pick up with a spoon or hold in your hand and is possible to explore with *all* your senses. Imagine that you have never seen it before. You are examining it for the first time and need to know all you can about it. Note any assumptions or expectations you might have about the object and the exercise itself.

1. Examine the object carefully with your eyes.
2. Examine the object carefully by touching it and exploring it as completely as possible, relying on tactile as well as visual perception.
3. Notice if there is any smell associated with the object. If so, examine it in different positions and distances as completely as you can. Is the smell constant, or does it change?
4. Listen to it. Are any sounds associated with it? Feel free to manipulate the object to see if and how that affects it.
5. Place it in your mouth, noticing all that involves. Notice where it is in your mouth. What taste is there, if any? How does it feel? What else do you notice? Examine it with your tongue and see

if you can bite into it. What happens? Stop after each bite (if it is food) until it disappears.

Jot down what you observed, including anything you may have learned about this experience. Pause and reflect on what you discovered about yourself and this process of paying attention. How might you use this information?

· · · · · · · · · · ·

5 / Befriending the Body

Discovering What's Right Rather than Wrong

The old gray mare, she ain't what she used to be, ain't what she used to be . . .
—*Folk song*

Recently, I found myself humming, "The old gray mare, she ain't what she used to be, ain't what she used to be . . ." No, I ain't what I used to be. My body is aging, and I don't leap up from a sitting position like as I used to do. The years and chemotherapy have affected me, yet I am happy that I have a body. I like my body. I respect how it has taken me through some difficult times. I can walk, swallow, and breathe without an oxygen mask. How wonderful. I do not take this for granted. I haven't always been able to do these things, and I have no idea how long such freedom will last. Remembering this truth helps me maintain perspective when I'm having trouble rising from my chair.

Everything is always changing, including us. Each breath that we feel and follow as it enters and leaves the body is a reminder of our aliveness and the preciousness of each moment.

I treasure my body and do my best to take care of it. I eat consciously and savor every bite, including samples of the three pies that were on the table at Thanksgiving. I really, really enjoyed the tartness of the cherry, the smooth texture of the pumpkin, and the sweetness of the apple. If I didn't appreciate and enjoy the taste of every bite, why bother? I have had to adapt to the physical changes in my body due to aging and chemotherapy. Sometimes the song "I'm a Little Teapot, Short and Stout" pops into my head, but I smile and do my best to accept my body as it is.

As for my little teapot "steaming up," how great that the energy of my mindfulness practice keeps me hot and boiling away. It's another reminder that I'm here and living life. Please let me be of service; "pour me out!"

Listening to my body tells me how to pace myself and maintain energy so I can do what is meaningful without depleting myself. Since I tire easily, I sometimes have to take a nap or limit the amount of work I do. It is not always easy or simple to say "No" and acknowledge fatigue, but limits must be respected. I'm deluding myself and failing to help anyone else if I don't pay attention to the messages my body is sending me. As my mother would say, I've learned this the hard way.

Not long before my sixtieth birthday, I was on a Metta retreat (*metta* in the ancient Pali language means "loving-kindness") not far from my home in Massachusetts. This is a retreat that cultivates kindness and compassion toward all beings in the world, including ourselves. For five days, I repeated to myself, "May I be safe and protected. May I be happy. May I be healthy. May I live with ease." But one morning, I became aware of a sharp pain in my side. I noted the pain, felt the different sensations, and kept repeating the same phrases. I returned to the meditation hall, sat, and continued saying the phrases to myself throughout the afternoon and evening. The pain did not abate, but I ignored it, even when it woke me up in the middle of the night. The next day, still in pain, I continued repeating the phrases to myself. My concentration was strong, and I was able to bear the sensations, which were now more intense and continuous. I did not want to leave the retreat or acknowledge something could be seriously wrong with me. It wasn't until a staff member saw that I could not bend down to tie a shoelace and suggested that I go to a nearby clinic that I acknowledged that I needed to see a doctor. Even after I was examined at a nearby clinic, I hesitated to pack my belongings. The clinic doctors didn't know what was causing the pain, which had now become acute. It never occurred to me that it could be caused by a recurrence of lymphoma. I called my husband, a primary care physician, who told me to go to the emergency room, but I said, "After the dharma talk," and stubbornly waited in pain until it was over.

Looking back, I think how paradoxical it was that this particular retreat was intended to cultivate care and kindness. By ignoring my symptoms and hoping they would go away, I was doing just the opposite. My denial was so strong that when I finally left the retreat center and drove myself home (it never occurred to me to ask for help or that it could be dangerous to drive), I left the sheets on the bed, hoping this was something simple and I could return before the retreat ended.

That evening, I had a CT scan in the ER, and we discovered the pain was caused by the cessation of blood to a tumor. It was lymphoma and a discernible mass, and it needed to be removed immediately. I had surgery the next day and humbly donated my sheets to the meditation center.

Eight years have passed since that time, but the memory is still vivid. Concentration helps us be mindful, but it doesn't automatically bring wisdom. That only comes through the commitment to face what is true; only then can we manage it wisely. In my case, I wanted so badly *not* to have a recurrence of lymphoma that I deluded myself and didn't listen to the wisdom of my body, which was saying to me, "Take care of this!"

This experience has humbled me. It has taught me the consequences of wanting things to be different than they are. As you do the body scan that follows this chapter or that's available for download at www.shambhala.com/BeingWell, allow yourself to feel your body *as it is.* Do your best *not* to try to change anything or make it go away. This practice enhances control and manageability of symptoms through accepting and directly meeting what is present without the filter of likes and dislikes. (Those distractions will be there, but you can learn from them; simply note "pleasant" or "unpleasant" as they cross your mind, or just say, "Thinking," to yourself and observe the effect in the body.) I will always respect the power of denial and the delusion that comes from holding on to what we want rather than accepting what we have. It's good to be able to meet what we label "pain" by breathing with it and softening into it, but it still needs to be addressed. My discounting of my pain was false. It is equally false to be overly concerned when something feels a little different. How many times have you felt a twinge and panicked, thinking it was cancer? Or perhaps you feel a tightness in your chest and think you're having a heart attack. I am not suggesting that you ignore these symptoms—on the contrary, have them checked out by your doctor. But they may also be caused by fear and anxiety.

Lenny, an intelligent and skilled professional, heard that I—like him—was living with lymphoma. He knew that I did training in mindfulness-based stress reduction and called to ask if he could have a session with me. He reported that every little twinge suggested that he was having a recurrence of cancer. He was in remission and feeling healthy and strong, but no matter how hard he tried, he could not stop worrying. This was affecting his work and his family life. When he came into my office, he was miserable and miserable about being miserable, convinced he *should* be able to control his thoughts. Though he was successful at helping others, he felt like a failure at helping himself.

As he sat across from me, I observed a middle-aged man, well groomed and articulate but so agitated that he was barely able to stay in his seat. His speech was rapid, and he began to sweat as he told me how he kept trying to stop thinking that he was dying.

I listened and nodded sympathetically, knowing that this is a common phenomenon once cancer has been diagnosed. We live with the fear it will happen again.

"You can't will these thoughts away," I told him. "You can name the thought 'worry,' and you can even count the number of times it comes into your head and time how long it lasts, but you can't force it to disappear. Only by accepting that this is simply the way your mind works can the thought lose its energy and dissipate. What is the evidence that your feelings are true?"

There was no evidence, and it was novel to Lenny to consider examining the thought itself, acknowledge it, and observe what would happen next. He had been trying to avoid the thought or talk himself out of it. I know from experience that this never works. I asked him if he would be willing to investigate the thought by noticing when it occurred, how often, and for how long.

Lenny said, "Yes," and I assigned that task as homework.

We then turned to that moment, there in my office. I had him bring awareness to his breath by putting his hand on his belly. I knew Lenny was a thinker; he had a wonderful mind, and it helped him to succeed professionally. Now, though, he needed to pay attention to his body—his whole body, not just his twinges and areas of concern. It was important that he *feel* his breath rather than think about it. I knew taking him out of his head and his intrusive thoughts would be helpful. After a few minutes of observing his breath, the movements of his belly and chest began to slow and become more rhythmic. He continued feeling each breath as it moved his hand up and down for about five minutes. The more he relaxed, feeling the breath rising and falling in the region of his belly, the quieter he became. I'm sure his mind was still busy, but now he was using breath to anchor his attention and creating a home he could return to again and again. His breath was serving as a reminder to observe his thinking rather than getting lost in it and mistaking his fears for reality.

The more we cultivate breath as an anchor of attention, the more it can be a place to rest, stop, and renew our intentions and perspective. Repeatedly returning our attention to it when we realize we are lost in a stream of thoughts trains the mind to be present. It focuses the mind so we can ride the currents of our emotions as we observe our breathing. The breath continues to send nutrients to our cells, cleanse our system, and is a reminder that we are still here.

. . . .

STOP

Take a moment to honor your body and appreciate that it allows you to be here. You can bring attention to your breath, letting it be as it is. If you like, as you breathe in, you can feel the renewal that comes with the inhalation; as you breathe out, feel the release of toxins, worries, and fears.

. . . .

The Body Scan

Mr. Duffy lived at a little distance from his body.

—James Joyce

Participants in the MBSR program are asked to practice a body scan every day for two and a half weeks, forty-five minutes a day. This is not about "doing" a scan, but rather about receiving attention and care. It is best done lying in a supine position, supported and resting on a bed, a recliner, or perhaps a mat on the floor. It is best to enter into the scan without striving for something to happen. This encourages a real letting go and a deep surrender and release.

Most people, like Mr. Duffy in Joyce's *Dubliners,* do not inhabit the body. We spend much of our time in our heads, even if we exercise regularly, practice yoga, and spend time on our appearance. For this reason, the scan begins at the toes. We also spend a lot of time focusing on the left foot, so don't be surprised when you hear this instruction. This is to help the mind focus on a body part that is usually neutral and not charged with emotion. This approach helps in quieting and calming; when a strong sensation arises, you will have some experience in noting sensation (or the lack thereof) and be able to use the breath to breathe with it.

In the MBSR program, we used to suggest participants imagine having a blowhole like a whale's at the top of their head through which energy cycled through their body, but we discovered there is no need to imagine a blowhole to feel the whole body and the breath flowing through it. Feeling your breath as it moves through your body—and your body as a whole—is enough. Nor is there is any need to feel perfect to be whole. We have done this scan with people in wheelchairs and amputees. It is done in prisons and many widely divergent settings. It is a powerful meditation that brings mind and body together. It can be comforting and soothing.

I like bringing compassion and affectionate attention to the body, especially parts that are tender or sensitive. I sometimes find it helpful to imagine the body bathed in light, with energy entering it from above, below, and all around. The scan can also bring forth old memories or disturbing thoughts that demand your attention. At those times, it can be a leap of faith to know that by allowing them to enter your awareness and bring them forth into consciousness, you are connecting to what you need for healing to take place. Paradoxically, breathing with pain, either emotional or physical, can break us open into wellness by helping us drop defenses that are no longer useful. We are connecting to what we need to be free. If the pain becomes too intense, it is useful to open your eyes, listen to sounds, or perhaps move around. You are in charge. It is skillful to have as many ways of coping as possible. Through the scan, we cultivate the ability to listen to and learn from the body rather than trying to make anything special happen.

Mary, a breast cancer patient, began doing the body scan when she came to me during chemotherapy. She found the words of the scan, its tone, and its phrasing soothing. She did it, not only during her treatment, but also at home when she was feeling anxious and sick from the chemo's side effects. It helped her when she was nauseous and taught her to relax rather than tense and struggle uselessly. It also enabled her to ask her doctor to reevaluate her medications as she realized it was neither wise nor necessary to feel that she had to "tough it out." Mindfulness and medicine go well together, but one is not a substitute for the other. Listening to her body kept Mary's fear under control; she had been diagnosed with stage IV cancer and had had surgeries as well as radiation. She lived with the knowledge that she might need to switch drugs and treatment at any time, as the cancer could be very aggressive.

Mary planned her sessions with me for when she had energy, working around her chemotherapy schedule, two weeks on and one week off. She was becoming skilled at predicting her periods of highest energy and how to pace herself. By listening to her body, she knew when to stop and take a nap and when to plan outings. She was practicing being more realistic—and less anxious—about what she could and could not do. Around the holidays, Mary realized she would need a longer period between treatments so she could visit her son, who lived some distance away. She wanted to enjoy her time with him, and she knew a long car ride would be uncomfortable and tire her out. She asked her doctor if she could safely give herself extra time between treatments to have more energy for the drive.

Mary and I discussed how she could care for her body on her trip. This meant being honest with her family (and herself). For example, she told her husband that she would need to make frequent stops to get out of the car and go to the bathroom. We also explored how to enhance her comfort in the car by bringing a pillow so she could lie down in the backseat. She decided to take her CD with guided meditations and earphones so she could listen without distractions. She had used the CD enough times to know that it would be beneficial in helping her relax.

When Mary returned from the trip, she was very tired but happy. Her resourcefulness and commitment to family and to self-care had helped her get through the difficulty of the journey. She had already endured surgery, radiation, and many bouts of chemotherapy. Most important, she felt empowered. She knew she could manage pain if it arose and rely on her judgment to rest or ask for help if she felt it was required.

The first CD I made for cancer patients didn't contain a body scan. I thought it might be too disturbing to spend time bringing awareness into the body when it was already grappling with pain and illness. Instead, I found the opposite to be true. Rather than making people feel betrayed, moving from toes to head with awareness seemed to help them make friends with their body. This was as true on the transplant unit and in ambulatory settings as in a stress reduction classroom.

Guided Body Scan Meditation

As you do this scan, it is helpful to remember that everything that arises also passes away. Let your willingness to pay attention and listen to your body inform you and guide you without any expectations of what should happen. Please don't judge yourself if negative thoughts arise. Note them. They will pass. As soon as you discover you are lost in these thoughts, all you need to do is return your attention to the body, remembering to do so tenderly, with compassion and love. Notice what is not painful as well as any strong sensation that you label "pain." Stay with a sensation as long as possible and observe how it changes. You can always open your eyes, listen to sounds, or consciously change position. May this be an adventure of love, peace, and self-discovery.

To start, bring your awareness to your breath and let it rest in an area where it is easy to observe its effect on the body. If you like, you can rest your hand on your belly, imagining the belly is like a balloon filling with air and rising on the in-breath and falling, like a balloon deflating, on the out-breath. Simply notice; do not try to change your breath in any way, but bring awareness to the motion of breathing. You can note whether the breath is slow or fast, even or irregular. Remember not to judge what is happening; simply observe.

When you're ready, let your eyes close. Mentally sweep through the body, letting yourself experience the body as a whole, and imagine that each breath is filling it with light and love. Notice the parts of the body you can feel easily, others that may be tender, and those you can barely discern; notice when you want to push away or close down, as well as when you want to linger longer. When your attention wanders, simply bring it gently but firmly back to the body.

When you are ready, allow your awareness to move gently and caringly down the body into your foot on the left side. If you are short of time, you can do both feet together; however, do not rush this process. Slowly connect to your foot, beginning with the toes, moving into the heel, the sole, the arch, and the top of the foot, appreciating that it has served you well through the years. You can let the foot (feet) dissolve in your awareness and direct your attention into the ankle. If there is a vivid experience in another area of the body, you can note it and compassionately bring your attention to it, and then when you are ready, you can let it go and return to where you were. Simply notice, breathing with the sensation and softening into it with loving care.

Repeat this process of noting, opening, and softening into whatever arises through the body. Move from the feet through the following sequence: ankle, lower leg, knee, thigh, and into the pelvic area (groin, genitals, buttocks, and hips), spine, lower back, middle back, upper back, shoulder, upper arm, elbow, lower arm, wrist, hand, fingertips, abdomen, diaphragm, chest, throat, neck, and head. Beginning with the jaw, move up through the face from mouth to ears to nose to eyes to eyebrows to the point between the eyebrows to the forehead and into the scalp.

Let yourself rest in the sensations of the moment, releasing tension and worries with the out-breath and bringing in a sense of wellness, caring, and renewal with the in-breath. If you like, when you have finished scanning the body, you can imagine an opening at the crown of the head through which energy enters, and imagine this energy traveling through the body as a whole and bringing with it what you need. Let it caress the body with love and attention and release what needs to go. Imagine energy moving in through the soles of your feet and up through the entire body, and releasing at the crown of the head, then coming back in through the crown and out through the soles of your feet. You may do this body scan as many times as you wish, knowing that each time you do, you are taking an active part in your own wellness and healing.

6 / Meeting Pain

The truth that many people do not understand is that the more you try to avoid suffering, the more you suffer, because smaller and more insignificant things begin to torture you in proportion to your fear of being hurt.

—*Thomas Merton*

Pain can wear us down and tire us out, but it need not defeat us, depending on how we meet it. It may seem like an oxymoron to be at peace when in pain. Pain can be so direct, so immediate, that it fills all the spaces in our mind, forcing us to notice it and understand its message. Sometimes we can distract ourselves from it, but other times it is unavoidable. Yet the greater our repertoire of response and the more willing we are to befriend and understand how we relate to the sensations that we label as "pain," the more control we have in managing it.

A patient of mine tells me she has learned to "obey" pain. It tells her when she needs to rest or push herself to build up her muscles now that she's stronger. In the past, her familiarity with her body led her to suspect that something was wrong. It helped her go to her doctor, who validated her concern and discovered a new cancer, which he then successfully treated before it had spread widely. Listening to the body and trusting its messages comes with practice. Treatment for cancer or other serious diseases can have side effects, some dangerous, others normal. It takes some objectivity to be able to discern when to pay attention and get help and when to make friends with the aftereffects of treatment. Another of my patients underwent radiation to treat a brain tumor and has learned which signs to heed as well as how and when to reassure herself that the cancer is not recurring. She also has steroid-induced diabetes. The steroids saved her life, but now she needs to monitor her blood sugar levels. She must listen to the signals her body sends to know when and what to eat.

Meeting pain requires calm attention. We learn to witness and observe in a nonreactive, "nondoing" mode that can feel counterintuitive. The body registers danger, and we are hardwired to fight or flee. This is not always possible. Distraction works some of the time, and medication—monitored by a skilled professional—definitely helps. Palliative care is available and important; no one needs to endure pain if it can be alleviated. It is merciful to use medication under a doctor's supervision. I don't think I could have made it through my stem cell transplant and surgeries without the help of pain relievers. Even with medication, I was very sick and couldn't avoid pain. But I know I didn't suffer psychologically. My mouth was filled with sores and I couldn't eat, but I enjoyed the popsicles they had on the transplant unit. I focused on the sky outside my window and spent hours noticing how it changed. I appreciated the comfort of a back rub and my caring friends. I enjoyed talking to the nurses and staff on the unit. I focused on the present moment and lived in it. I didn't feel there was a choice. It was the only way to keep from suffering and be alive.

At one critical point, I remember lying in bed and feeling the softness of the mattress and the warmth of the blanket over me. I could do nothing but focus on my breath, breath by breath, sinking into each one. Any slight tension, any bit of struggle stopped me from breathing. I surrendered. I could not talk, I could not move; all I could do was lie back, sink into the mattress, and receive breath. I could only be open to each breath, slowly, one at a time. Inhale, exhale: that was my world. I sensed people in the room, felt their presence, their care, and their worry. But my job was to let be—no fighting, no doing. To just let my breath come and go without any volition. I remember hearing the sound of children outside the room and thinking, "If I die, it's OK. Life goes on."

In-breath, out-breath, peace. It was effortless.

Years later, I visited my oncologist, who told me that my lungs had been almost totally filled with fluid. She and the team were considering putting me on a respirator. My husband had been told not to go to work and to sit by my side and try to be calm. At the time, I had no idea that the time *after* stem cells are reintroduced into the body and before the immune system has had a chance to mature was perilous, nor did I know that I had pneumonia. What I remember is a sense of surrender and feeling peaceful. I wondered why people seemed worried. I wasn't being brave or courageous. I didn't consciously say to myself, "Let go" or "Let be." It just made sense to do the only thing I could do—trust what would be and breathe. I also remember feeling surrounded by love.

There is no formula for meeting pain, softening into it rather than struggling against it. If you are a person of faith, faith helps. Experience helps. Knowing your body and being able to interpret sensations wisely comes with practice.

Eliza has been treated with chemotherapy successive times for more than one cancer and has been repeatedly hospitalized. She has had a series of upper respiratory infections and pneumonia. Even a cold can be dangerous for her. I asked her how she manages to maintain perspective. She told me that she has learned to discern which symptoms to address. "If a cough persists, or I wake in the night feeling poorly," she says, "I call the doctor. Otherwise, I talk to myself. I'm not going to get too excited about it. I know my doctor is sharp; he keys in on what is important and accessible. He communicates with me." Remembering how she has come through many previous difficulties, she has learned to reassure herself that she need not worry unduly.

Cultivating patience and calm makes a difference. So does living in the present moment. Thich Nhat Hahn, a Vietnamese teacher of meditation, wrote a little poem called a *gatha*:

Breathing in I calm,
Breathing out I smile,
Dwelling in the present moment
It is a precious moment.

It is normal to worry. Once something bad has happened, we know it can happen again, which is why it is helpful to bring ourselves back to the present moment and our direct experience. Congratulate yourself every time you stop yourself from floating away, lost in the past or fabricating a future reality that doesn't exist. You are cultivating an ability to engage in a more realistic appraisal of what you need.

Such surrender doesn't come easily; it requires the effort of practice. Every time you notice tension in the body and anchor your attention back to the here and now (through your breath, a sound, the position of your feet, the scene outside your window, or an object nearby), you are strengthening your mindfulness muscle. Can you notice the difference between the contraction of fear and the soft, open awareness of acceptance? The effort to be mindful and surrendering to what is—gliding into a sensation with your breath rather than struggling against it—enhances relaxation and ease. This alters the experience of pain rather than stopping it. Expecting cessation and striving to make it happen will only perpetuate contraction and tensing.

* * * * * * * * * *

Let go. Allow. Trust. Breathing with the sensations that you are feeling rather than fighting them alters your experience so you can calm and rest.

* * * * * * * * * *

Discover for yourself how it is to STOP when you notice you're struggling. Gently practice meeting pain and relaxing into it, sensation by sensation. Do it only as long as you can, then distract yourself, push a button for a nurse if you're in the hospital, change your position or move, get some support, or listen to the audio meditations. Please remember to be compassionate to your self; know that you are doing your best and this is hard. Don't expect to like what you are feeling, but be patient. There will be a change.

* * * * * * * * * *

Being understanding and kind helps.

* * * * * * * * * *

By noticing where you are and what you are doing, thinking, and feeling and stopping to observe without judging what you observe, you will be connecting to what you need. Trust this process and discover for yourself what helps you. Give yourself permission to STOP and receive the space and time you need to recover and calm. You can challenge yourself to STOP and notice when you are trying to change the unchangeable. What does it feel like to let go of striving to make something happen? How do you discriminate between what is pointless to try to change and what is worth the effort?

If you have begun the body scan, you may have noticed that the instructions say, "Do not try too hard to relax; this will just cause more tension." The instructions make sense but are not easy to execute because we *want* to feel good and avoid pain. In the mindfulness-based stress reduction program at the Center for Mindfulness, participants are asked to do the body scan daily for three weeks. Many of these people come because they want relief from pain and to learn how to cope with it better. Consistently, in my experience and those of other teachers, people report that they hate doing the body scan. They ask why they should do it. "It only makes me notice my pain more," they complain. Pain like muscle tension or joint pain that may have been under the radar until they stopped and slowed comes into awareness as well. "Yes," we say. "How interesting. How wonderful. You've been paying attention."

It is humbling to notice how we react to what we label "pain." It takes effort to pause and acknowledge the strain and state of mind—usually one of frustration, fear, or desire—that intensify and cause pain. We are surrendering to the truth of habits of mind that are well entrenched and automatic. To breathe with sensations that we label as "pain" and soften into them, meeting each sensation breath by breath and sensation by sensation, requires trust and struggle. We don't know if it will help us when we have to practice experiencing a belly that is soft rather than tense. We must feel what it is to meet pain and soften into it. This is effort driven by intention and a willingness to persevere. Let's call it "right effort," the kind that comes from your intention to be caring, kind, and compassionate to yourself as you observe and *do not judge yourself*. It is useful to remember your intention at these times. I recommend stopping here for a minute before you proceed.

· · · · · · · · · · ·

STOP

Stop!
Take a breath.
Open and observe what this moment is bringing.
Proceed.

· · · · · · · · · · ·

Reflection: What Does It Mean to Surrender?

What is the meaning of surrender for you? An image that comes to me when I think of surrender is of floating. I imagine myself letting go of all worries and fears and allowing myself to be held in the warmth of the water in a crystal clear pond, a sanctuary hidden from view and protected by majestic evergreens. I see the tops of the trees surrounding the pond and admire the green of the trees reflected in the blue of the lake. I am lying on my back, gently swaying as I gaze up at the sky. White cirrus clouds are slowly moving through the expanse of sky, and I feel at peace. As I open my eyes and return to my room, this sense of peace lingers with me, and I am grateful to be alive. Do you have an image that represents the peace of letting go, of surrender?

7 / Accepting Change

When you are through changing, you are through.

—*Bruce Barton*

I am sure to grow old.
I cannot avoid aging.
I am sure to become sick.
I cannot avoid sickness.
I am sure to die.
I cannot avoid death.
All things dear and beloved to me
are subject to change and separation.
I am the owner of my actions;
I will become the heir of my actions.

—*Anguttara Nikaya*

Every now and then something pivotal happens in our lives by which we measure time, a marker event such as 9/11, a marriage or divorce, a birth or death, or a diagnosis such as cancer. I've divided my own time into precancer and post–stem cell transplant. The time is marked not by age but by changes in my world. Precancer, mortality was a given intellectually, but after my diagnosis, I knew it in my heart, head, and gut. Death became a part of my awareness, and I could no longer delude myself into believing that illness and loss happened to others but not to me. When I was young, I had a sister who died shortly after she was born. This changed our family constellation, but I was too young to comprehend the effect it had on me until years later. Both of my parents died of cancer, but I could accept that, even though I mourned their loss. However, confronting my own death changed my view of myself; suddenly I was vulnerable and uncertain about my future. Who was I now? I did not want to be seen only as a cancer patient. The rhythm of my life changed. My time was now filled with doctors' appointments and managing the effects of chemotherapy rather than being a professional. I was no longer teaching patients but being a patient.

In this kaleidoscope of change, I struggled to find a fulcrum on which to rest. I was determined to see if it really was true, as we told the people in our stress reduction classes, that attitude makes a difference and suffering can be relieved. I was determined to do what I could to manage my feelings. My intention not to suffer was strong, but accepting the unacceptable—at least at first—was daunting. To cope, I had to acknowledge what had changed. To manage all the thoughts and feelings of my new reality, I had to accept what was real. This did *not* mean I had to like it. Indeed, it is the belief that acceptance means approval that prevents us from truly acknowledging whatever is causing us to suffer. In reality, each change can create new resistance and force us to dig deep down to find the strength to adapt again to altered conditions.

A woman I know who does hospice work is familiar with the changes that occur as a person approaches death, but she was unprepared when she learned that her nephew had jumped over a three-foot wall and landed, not on the grass as he had expected, but on a concrete floor twenty-five feet down. His pelvis was broken, and bones in his legs were shattered.

When she went to visit him in the hospital, she found him suffering from self-blame in addition to his injuries. "If only," he kept telling her. "If only I hadn't jumped over that wall."

She told him to leave the past behind. "You didn't hit your head," she said. Noting what did not happen, what could have been even worse, helped both her and him maintain perspective. It is not yet known how much mobility he will have, and it will take time and effort for him to adapt to his new circumstances. He needs strength, faith, and support, not regret. His feelings will not vanish immediately, but they can be held with compassion. Then acceptance can follow, and with it, healing.

. . . .

To accept change, we need to accept thoughts and feelings as well as our resistance to an altered life.

. . . .

. . . .

STOP

Let's take a breath and pause for a moment. Can you name the changes that you are experiencing? Which ones do you view as difficult or destabilizing? Are you thrown off balance? How? What do you feel in your body as you contemplate this situation?

There is no right or wrong, good or bad. Whatever emerges, including your reactions, simply note it. Let yourself be aware of what enters your awareness, noting both acceptance and resistance.

What positive changes have you experienced? What is your reaction to them? What do you notice in your body in this contemplation?

You can do this exercise in your head, but I recommend writing it down quickly and spontaneously without any censoring.

Changes/Responses (note thoughts, feelings, and sensations):

_____

_____

_____

_____

_____

_____

_____

_____

_____

. . . .

. . . .

STOP

Now that you have completed this exercise, give yourself some time to refocus and settle the mind. Allow yourself to take a breath, letting your attention rest with your breathing for a few minutes. As you do so, you can open your eyes and look around you. Can you feel your feet? What is the position of your body? If there is a window nearby, you can observe the scene outside your room. You can also observe the room you are in and let your eyes rest on the objects there. When you are ready, let your eyes close and return your attention to the next inhalation and exhalation. Do this for a minimum of five minutes.

After you are finished, I recommend rereading what you have written. Do you notice any changes in your reactions as you revisit the changes you have named? Would you like to add or delete anything? How much of what you've written do you wish hadn't happened? Where are the areas of resignation and negativity? Is there sadness or regret? Is there calm? Has your level of acceptance changed? Are you able to read what you have written with objectivity?

Acceptance is a process that happens with intention and in time. How do you experience acceptance? What words would you use to describe it?

· · · · · · · · · ·

What Contributes to Your Acceptance of Changes in Your Life?

Change can happen in a flash, but acceptance is a process. I asked a patient of mine who had recently recovered from serious surgery for esophageal cancer how she accepts the fact that she no longer has an esophagus. She can eat only small amounts of food and often experiences gastric distress. She replied, "I have to. It's the only choice I have."

We both laughed as she spoke, but I know that this acceptance hasn't come without struggle or mourning. She is still adjusting to the change in her life. Each time she eats, she is reminded that she is no longer the same and worries that she could have a recurrence of cancer. My patient has a good sense of humor and a strong support system that help her adapt to life without an esophagus. She is thankful to be alive. Gratitude now puts her gastric distress into perspective, but as she was going through the stress of diagnosis, surgery, and treatment, she used every resource she had to cope with her fear and pain. This included the support of friends and medical care. Her husband kept a blog, and after she recovered, her daughter made a video of her journey. This helped each of them as well as others. There was a reciprocity of support and caring that extended beyond the individual to the family and their extended community. Adapting to change is not automatic. It takes effort, time, space, and support.

Relationships change in the face of illness. Acquaintances may be more comfortable with the you who is ill than people who have been close to you. Everyone reacts differently; every member of the family is changed when someone is diagnosed with cancer. The best and the worst can manifest during times of crisis, and responses shift depending on the nature and severity of illness as well as circumstances, personalities, and age. I think it is wise to use available resources, visiting nurses, social workers, and counselors as well as your established support system. Nothing stays the same. Neither can you.

An exercise I've used to facilitate acceptance is adapted from a Tibetan meditation called *Tonglen*. In it, we let ourselves feel the pain of another (or our own) on an in-breath and—if desired—give the pain a color, a shape, and even a texture or weight. The pain is fully experienced on the inhalation and, in the pause before the exhalation, converted to light and released. Letting it in and bringing it close helps us know it. We release fear by facing fear. We release hurt and worry by meeting hurt and worry. Breath by breath, it is converted and released.

I have also done a similar exercise with soap bubbles. To demonstrate change (and the temporal nature of thoughts), I took a bottle of bubbles and a wand to my stress reduction class at the Dana Farber Cancer Institute. Everyone in the class was in different stages of cancer, some in treatment and others in posttreatment, and I asked them to think of something troubling as they dipped their wands into the soapy solution. People laughed, but they grew serious as they allowed negative thoughts to form in their minds. They then carefully took a thought, held it for a moment, and blew it out into the soapy solution, watching as it formed bubbles of different shapes and hues and floated away. We all watched silently as, one by one, each bubble burst open and disappeared. I now keep a giant wand and pan on reserve. There is always something that can be troubling—and it is always possible to let it go.

Do you believe it is possible to be accepting of what you resist? Can you let it go?

· · · · · · · · · ·

• STOP • Refocus • Breathe • Feel Your Feet • Look at the Sky • Smile • Remember Your Intention

· · · · · · · · · ·

One of my teachers, Joseph Goldstein, has talked about the use of attention and gathering the joy of concentration. We can find peace and respite from pain by remembering that it is possible to stop and shift our focus to a neutral object or one that connects us to what is here with us now—the sky, a sip of water, a smile. This paying attention and being mindful, breath by breath and step by step, takes intention. Adding patience, perseverance, and kindness to our intention helps steady and calm the mind, making it easier to maintain perspective and let go.

When the mind is calm, it is easier to see clearly and maintain perspective, *but* this requires time and space. We cannot talk ourselves into acceptance. It requires a very deep surrender to acknowledge that we cannot change the unchangeable and to let go of the "if onlys."

Take a moment and fill in this sentence:

"If only _____, then _____."

For example: If only I didn't have cancer, then my life would be perfect.

"If only _____, then _____."

"If only _____, then _____."

"If only _____, then I would be accepting of _____."

Now imagine what it could be like if you could let go of these "if onlys." Would you be happier? Would you feel more peaceful?

· · · · · · · · · ·

The calmness of inner peace is the antithesis of confusion, the antidote to hurt, and the salve of healing discomfort.

· · · · · · · · · ·

When I was ill, I had to accept that I wasn't accepting. I had to give it space and time. So I meditated, found inspirational readings, carried colored pencils and a notebook with me to jot down feelings and thoughts, found funny movies and entertaining books, and was thankful for the caring people in my life.

What helps you? Mindfulness points the way if you are open to its insights.

Reflection: Acceptance

With a partner, take turns asking, "What does *acceptance* mean for you?" The person who asks the question listens without speaking and, when the responder finishes, says, "Thank you," and then asks the question again. Do this for three to four minutes and then pause and silently bring your attention to your breath. After a minute, switch roles. When you have both done this reflection, pause again and then discuss what you have learned.

8 / Anxiety

Anxiety is the hand maiden of creativity.
   —*T. S. Eliot*

Love looks forward, hate looks back, anxiety has eyes all over its head.
   —*Mignon McLaughlin*

Mindfulness is paradoxical. Everything has at least two sides, the good and the bad—and of course, all that lies in between. Anxiety can be useful as a warning that something is not quite right or as an impetus, as T. S. Eliot suggests, to doing something that will be beneficial. There can be anticipatory anxiety, the excitement that gives us energy for tasks such as preparing for a test, or anxiety that is so severe that we are paralyzed. Anxiety in moderate doses is positive. I get somewhat anxious before a talk, and it spurs me on. It gives me the boost I need to be prepared and dissipates once I become absorbed in the task at hand. Too much, however, would affect my presentation and make me less coherent.

There are times when anxiety is unavoidable. I am always anxious before I have a new CT scan. I only relax after the doctor sees me and tells me its results. I find it easier to cope with a recurrence than worrying about it. I've learned to say to myself, "I'll get through this," and I know that I have (three times). I was *very* anxious before my stem cell transplant. I calmed once I was in the hospital. There was no other choice if I wanted to be well. On a moment-to-moment basis, reality is manageable; staying in my head and imagining what could happen is not. When things were really challenging (bad), I couldn't be anxious. My attention was focused on surviving, breath by breath. No one likes to be nauseous, but if you are, you can't be anxious; nausea absorbs all your attention. You don't need to contract and resist; this makes it worse. It makes much more sense to breathe with and soften into the spasms. This takes practice. It is counterintuitive *but worth practicing*. Each time you notice yourself breathing in response to tension rather than resisting, you are strengthening your ability to move with sensation, even the waves of nausea and the feelings that go with them. No one can tell you to do this; you must discover it for yourself. It takes courage to keep practicing when some of what you observe is fear, hurt, or anger.

Anxiety can overtake us, cloud our vision, accelerate our heart rates, jam our brains, and make us self-absorbed and miserable. Right? Exhale if this statement resonates with you—and please remember compassion. Anxiety is so common that I have actually found iPhone apps to control it. One features a picture of a leaf and a feather. You are asked to pair them as they rise and fall so they are on the same plane. This refocuses your attention, giving you a sense of control and slowing your breathing. I don't think you need a smartphone to do this. You can train yourself to use an object of attention that can help you refocus and slow your breath. I like feeling my feet, looking around and gazing at a neutral object, and remembering that this will pass. You can even choose to sing a favorite song.

On a bone marrow transplant unit, there are good reasons to be anxious. A transplant is a daunting procedure, and anything can happen, including death. When I was involved in the research project that brought mindfulness to patients undergoing stem cell transplants, we hoped that it would alleviate stress and anxiety. It was a large, four-year study of about 240 patients, who were randomly divided into three groups. One group worked with a mindfulness instructor, one group had a nurse educator, and another received regular care. As the consultant to this study, I was responsible for ensuring consistency and helping the instructors effectively communicate mindfulness.

It was more challenging than I had expected to introduce mindfulness to this population. The instructors were steeped in their own personal mindfulness practice. The nurses were all accustomed to giving concrete aid, like medication, to relieve suffering. They were dedicated, compassionate people with years of medical training and patient contact, but it was very hard for them not to "fix" the problem. I discovered that it was also challenging for them to trust that their ability to embody mindfulness was more potent in conveying its essence than their ability to describe it.

Strangely enough, the instructors were often more anxious than the patients they were teaching. Their feelings that it was important to follow the research procedure and "get it right" interfered with their own ability to be present. If a patient was sweating and breathing quickly, the instructor had to note "sweating and rapid breath" (anxiety) and help that patient bring attention to it, soften into it, and ride it out. Mindfulness has to make sense and be understood experientially, not just intellectually. There is no single way to describe it, no formula. Mindfulness is contextual and needs to fit each person and situation. When we discovered that the script we had prepared for the instructors to define mindfulness actually interfered with their ability to be mindful, we dropped it.

A sense of safety and calm is the antithesis of anxiety. In our study, the patients' first introduction to mindfulness came during phoresis. This is a procedure that extracts stem cells from the blood. (These cells are reinserted later to restart the immune system, which by then has been wiped out by intensive chemotherapy.) This is a time of high anxiety, and it is filled with uncertainty. It takes place before hospitalization. Imagine you may have traveled far from home; you are in a small, cramped, noisy room; and you are not sure that this procedure will be successful. A certain amount of stem cells are required for the transplant, and you may or may not have enough. You know that when you are eventually hospitalized, it is likely you will become quite ill, have fevers, be nauseated, and develop mouth sores. You will be isolated in a sterile environment and could die. Yet you have chosen to go through a stem cell transplant because you know cancer cells will be killed, and it can extend your life. Now a stranger comes into the phoresis room to see you. She is here to describe mindfulness and have you listen to meditations. You have agreed to participate in the study and learn about mindfulness because you hope it will be helpful—not just for you, but also for others.

Some patients in our study had heard of mindfulness, but most had not. At our initial meeting, we gave them an MP3 player and a CD they could use for the duration of the study. This CD was about 15 minutes long and included a body scan, a loving-kindness meditation, and practice in using the breath as an anchor of attention. An instructor sat with them and listened to the meditations along with them on another headset. This enabled the instructor to be in sync with the patients and answer any questions that arose. The intention was also to connect, saying in effect, "We're in this with you. Let us support you."

Mindfulness is present-focused and based on direct experience. It recognizes that this moment is our ground and worthy of attention. What is here for us now is all we have to work with, yet if there is something happening that we don't like, we tend to run from its reality. This response is normal, natural, and human. Sometimes it even works, but usually only on a temporary basis. I think it takes faith, trust, and courage to meet the moment and be willing to examine what it is bringing. Experiencing the relief that mindfulness brings comes only with practice. Softening into fear, anxiety, and pain can be a leap of faith.

Beneath anxiety lies fear: fear of loss, fear of change, fear of pain. All of these feelings are present when one is sick and facing a major procedure. The phoresis room was noisy and filled with people and machines. It was not a serene environment or conducive to calm. We wanted to do everything we could to gain the confidence of the people in our study and engage their curiosity and interest, as well as help them feel safe. We let them know we would always respect their wishes and that they were in charge of this intervention; they could either listen to the CD we brought them or not, as they wished.

As you may have discovered by now, beginning to practice and training the mind to calm by noting what arises takes determination and perseverance. In the beginning, it takes courage to pay attention to what flits through your awareness and believe it will be emancipating. Entering a new treatment can trigger all your defenses. It can be daunting to learn how your mind works and to discover the falsity of some of your beliefs and the ways you *think* you are helping yourself. We hoped that we could motivate transplant patients to use the meditations and enter into new experiences with greater acceptance and less resistance. It is helpful to know that everything changes, even vulnerability.

It also helps to know you don't have to be a victim of your own thoughts and suffer more than necessary, but you must discover this for yourself.

What helps you remember that nothing stays the same?

What reassures you that this (whatever you are struggling with) will pass?

What reminds you that you will manage and get through your difficulty?

What helps you know that the locus of control lies within you?

When you are sick, there is a lot to worry about in addition to your health. Finances can be a problem; there can be concerns about family members. You are no longer the person you used to be, so a sense of control needs to be reexperienced. Life is no longer the same.

My husband and I know that our life together will be divided into everything that happened before April 16, 2010—the date I was diagnosed with cancer—and everything that happens after it.

—*Entry from a patient's blog*

Of course, it's almost impossible not to worry during this time. Trying to talk yourself out of it will only make matters worse. Instead, take the plunge, feel what you're feeling. Allow it! Feel what it means to be anxious—the beating of your heart, the sweaty palms, the racing thoughts—*and* feel your feet. Focus on sound. Breathe with what arises moment by moment, and have faith that it will pass and you can regain your balance. Each time you do, it will be easier.

The instructors in the study I described reinforced this knowledge through their presence. They helped guide each person through the meditations and expanded them when they were with patients in their hospital rooms. These meditations were not used in place of medication; in fact, sometimes we urged a patient to ask for more medication to control nausea better or relieve pain. Yet each instructor who sat with a patient brought the intention to be accepting of whatever arose: fear, doubt, worry, joy, gratitude, and even laughter. Acceptance is key—and sometimes we need others to show us the way. It takes practice and determination to catch the mind at the beginning of a thought that can touch off a panic or anxiety attack and shift it from thought to direct experience. The instructors were with the patients for only a half hour at a time once or twice a week. The challenge was to bring awareness to the feel of the blanket or the coolness of an ice cube, the smile of a nurse or an aide, a photo on the table, and all the small wonders of everyday life.

Here are some comments from patients who participated:

"Sometimes I'd listen to the breath of the air and the wind blowing, and the calmness of the whole thing just put you in a different mindset. I found that very relaxing." (posthospitalization)

"In a way, I kind of let go of that frantic clinging to life, and I'm willing to go with the flow." (day two of hospitalization)

"I do find that mindfulness thing helpful, because it helps you to not reach for repression right away. It acknowledges that something is going on." (day ten of hospitalization)

"I don't knowingly practice now, but my approach to things is just a lot better, and I think that is a result of being more mindful overall." (posthospitalization)

My hope is that you, too, will do the meditations described in this book. As you read, the *moment* you recognize your heart beating rapidly, a tightening in your belly, and thoughts of doom and gloom, refocus, return to the here and now, feel your feet, clasp your hands, look about you, and remember—this will pass.

. . . .

Kindly practice, practice, practice, and keep practicing anchoring your attention in the here and now.

. . . .

There are many anchors of attention. You can use the breath; you can use the body as a whole, noting sensations, sounds, or images that are in your direct experience. Return to some words or phrases that you have used successfully to bring you into a state of relaxation. You can even sing to yourself, blaring out, "Anxiety, anxiety . . ." to your own tune. Exaggerate it. Shout it out! Ride its waves and let it pass. The waves may be choppy and the winds wildly blowing, but you will have spent time creating your own haven of ease by consistently doing any of the meditations here.

. . . .

In-breath . . . Out-breath. This will pass. . . . I am safe. I am alive. I am here.

. . . .

9 / Stress

The mind can make a heaven of hell, a hell of heaven.
  —*John Milton*

Aim always for your highest obtainable aim, but never put up resistance in vain.

Without stress, there would be no life.
  —*Hans Selye*

Hans Selye, the father of research on stress, coined the term *stress* in the 1950s. He defined it as a nonspecific response of the body to a demand. He was aware that demands could be good and bad, but both forced the body to adapt to change. Failure to do so over time led to exhaustion and disease. Selye's ability to be nonjudgmental and observe universal suffering with compassion has inspired me. My motto "Yes to life and all that's in it" is influenced by his work. Yes, I want to open to all that life can offer me, and yes, I want to be aware of what hinders and what helps me be open to it all—and, as the Serenity Prayer says, "have the wisdom to know the difference."

Richard Lazarus, a psychologist, looked at stress from a psychological perspective and defined it as "a particular relationship between the person and the environment that is *appraised* by the person as taxing or exceeding his or her resources and endangering his or her well-being" (1966, *Psychological Stress and the Coping Process*). The stressor is neutral; how we view it determines our reaction to it.

We can all agree that being sick is stressful. It affects us physiologically and psychologically. It is a crisis that the Chinese define as both danger and opportunity, because both depend on our perception of events and our appraisal of them.

Yesterday, I was at a memorial for my dear friend Stephanie, who died of breast cancer after many years in remission. She had planned the service before she died, instructing everyone to come in brightly colored clothes to celebrate her life. One friend danced to music; another friend read a poem Stephanie had written. We sat in silence, sending her blessings to ease her passing, and then we sang songs we knew she had loved. Family and friends spoke about her ability to appreciate who they were and to be caring and loving even as she was dying. Her daughter talked about the bliss her mother had experienced even as her body shut down. Stephanie had repeatedly told her, "It's not the life we are given but the courage we bring to it."

Stephanie was exceptional, but all of us, in our own way, have the ability to experience the peace and love that emanated from her through her last breath. I meditate for this reason. I know personally and through my observation of the wonderful patients I have worked with that such peace is possible. It is difficult and stressful but worthwhile, and it is up to us how we relate to the events in our lives. Are our actions satisfactory or unsatisfactory? What do we observe, and can we note what happens without judging?

Recently, my local public broadcasting station has been showing clips of babies as a promotion for a new program. The children are adorable, whether they are gurgling with delight and laughing or bawling loudly and demanding attention. They are all totally absorbed in what they are doing. Watching their natural curiosity and sense of exploration is fun and heartwarming. For babies, every moment holds the possibility for discovery and wonder. There are no preconceived expectations; everything is fresh and interesting. It brings joy to my heart to watch them.

Children are naturally and instinctively curious, while we adults must consciously remember to let go of the past and expectations before we can be as free to explore each moment as a child might. "Mindfulness" in Pali is *sati,* and its Sanskrit counterpart is *smriti,* which literally means "memory" or "to remember." The ability to be mindful requires ardor and vigor. It is not automatic. I must remember to be mindful. When I don't feel well, I find it helpful to have reminders that mindfulness is possible.

My friend Stephanie's life was mindfulness in action. Her life had been difficult, but she let herself maintain the curiosity and innocence of a child. "Sometimes she was too trusting," her husband said, "but what a joy it was to be with her. She was so filled with love and wonder."

The human brain has evolved to protect us from danger, and we are hardwired to survive by remembering the "bad" rather than the "good." We adults have to shed our layers of conditioning to be joyous and free. It takes courage to venture into the unknown and find the good in times of trouble. Stephanie acknowledged her illness; she did not flee from it, but she did not appraise it as emotionally disabling. It was a doorway for her to gain an even deeper appreciation of life and the people in it.

Anton Antonofsky, a sociologist who lived in the United States and Israel, was also interested in resilience. Studying women in menopause, some of whom had survived the Holocaust, he was surprised to discover how healthy these women were in comparison to a sample of women who had not experienced any significant trauma. As a result of this observation, he began to examine the characteristics of people who were successful in managing stress. He called this phenomenon *salutogenesis*. Elements of salutogenesis include *manageability,* the belief that you have the skills or ability, the support, the help, or the resources necessary to take care of things and that they are manageable and within your control; *meaningfulness,* the belief that things in life are interesting and a source of satisfaction; and *coherence,* the belief that there is good reason or purpose to care about what happens and that you are able to make sense of it.

When my father was diagnosed with cancer and I was his caregiver, I remember taking him to the hospital and seeing a posted sign that read as follows:

What Cancer Cannot Do

Cancer is so limited—
It cannot cripple love,
It cannot shatter hope,
It cannot corrode faith,
It cannot destroy peace,
It cannot kill friendship,
It cannot suppress memories,
It cannot silence courage,
It cannot invade the soul,
It cannot steal eternal life,
It cannot conquer the spirit.

Initially, I thought, "Yes, it can." I didn't know what to expect. My mother had suffered so much before she died from lung cancer that

I expected the same with my father. Later, I discovered that he had expected to beat the cancer. When he understood he could not, his ability to treat it as an adventure and death as a new land to discover kept his spirit alive. His expectation colored his experience and influenced mine when I was diagnosed with lymphoma a few years later.

Researchers are now investigating how the brain registers stress as well as the effect of meditation and compassion on the brain. They are discovering the areas of the brain that influence our perception of events and how we truly are what we think. The more a negative behavior is repeated, the more it strengthens its neural pathway and the harder it is to modify; the opposite is also true. The way we view events and how we act have measurable effects. The biblical expression that we reap what we sow is based on empirical evidence. If we are willing to examine our actions and beliefs without bias, we can discover whether they are helpful or not. Believing in our ability to affect our own well-being, we empower ourselves to have it happen. That puts the locus of control inside us rather than leaving us dependent on conditions beyond our control. For this reason, much of the MBSR program focuses on strengthening our ability to be aware of our thoughts, feelings, and sensations with the intention of understanding. When we judge what we observe harshly, we are interrupting the mind's ability to be in balance. Noting our tendency for self-criticism is useful. The moment we catch ourselves in negative reflection, we can refocus our attention and let it drop away.

Thomas Merton wrote, "We have what we seek; we have it all the time; and if we give it time, it will make itself known to us." Every time we catch ourselves becoming lost in reactivity (an automatic knee-jerk reaction) and STOP, we are providing an opportunity to discover what is being sought: understanding and peace. When striving to change the unchangeable ceases, contentment arises. Pausing gives us the time to consider how we want to respond. This loosens the noose of old conditioning. It helps us gain perspective and connect to what is needed in that moment. The challenge—as we experience the wear and tear of a life that includes aging, illness, loss, and death—is to experience each moment afresh. This cannot be done by holding on to our past. Just as with a small child learning a new skill, we are rewarded when we are persistent.

. . . .

STOP

What do you perceive as stressful? What is your stress reaction? How would you prefer to respond?

. . . .

In writing about stress, I have felt stressed; the subject is so large and all-encompassing. As a patient of mine said, "Why should I tune in and examine my stressors? My major way of coping is to distract myself."

I agree: we don't need to wallow in stress. If we can avoid what troubles us, great! What do we do, however, when distraction doesn't work and the stress of our pain—emotional, physical, or both—is unavoidable? Sometimes avoidance perpetuates the problem. How can we find what we seek if we refuse to look?

There are times when our conditioning is such that we are overwhelmed and unaware that we can pause and restabilize. At those times, we go to our default position. We are all unique in our approach to life. I tend to be a plunger. My motto is "Go for it!" My husband is a plodder. He'll count the trees, while I see only the forest. We need each other. I can be speedy and make mindless mistakes, such as forgetting where I left my cell phone. He is slow but steady and very organized. I am stubborn and persevere in the face of obstacles. I see them as a challenge and don't like giving up. My husband tends to acknowledge defeat more quickly than I do. We are both correct—some of the time. There is no wrong way, only different styles and conditioning. Our individual approaches influence how we cope when we get sick. They define our default position. Acting differently takes effort and the repetition of practice. It also means admitting that our default position is just that: a habitual response that has been learned.

Geri has been living with cancer for a number of years. She was recently told that the cancer had spread through her body. She came to my office to learn how to cope with this news and decide how best to proceed. When she realized that death was not imminent and her situation became more normalized, she complained that she had no control over herself. She couldn't stop herself from eating chocolate when she felt lonely. She was filled with self-disgust and had a poor body image. This was an old pattern for her. Shamefacedly, she told me how she would leave the house to buy chocolate if there was none left and then finish the bag in one sitting. Her anger and frustration with herself defeated the pleasure of the chocolate and only made her feel worse. She yearned to have someone with her who cared for her and was still angry that her husband had left her many years ago. She has friends but is reluctant to reach out to them for support and isolates herself when she feels most alone.

It can feel counterintuitive to embrace a stressor. Intellectually, we can acknowledge its usefulness in understanding the conditioning that underlies our stress reactivity, but emotionally, it is challenging.

Being forgiving of and compassionate with ourselves as we investigate our appraisal of events will lead us down more productive paths.

Geri perceives herself to be unattractive and unlovable, but this is not true. She is a bright, intelligent, and attractive person. She has many people who would be happy to talk with her if only she could pick up the phone and call them. When she feels tired and depleted, her mind goes to its default position ("I'm not good enough") and fixates on her inadequacies rather than her strengths. This self-blame and low self-worth is old stuff and blocks her from moving on. This pattern of thought is so automatic and well established that it feeds her habit of uncontrolled eating. On some level, the familiarity of this habit is comforting, but it certainly doesn't accomplish what she wants or needs. In our sessions, I try to help her be compassionate with and forgiving to herself, but she is not yet ready to let go of her hurt and anger. She can tell me about it in a session, but she is still reluctant to find different ways to soothe herself and feel whole. Our work in therapy is not about controlling her eating of chocolate but about believing in her own self-worth. Seeds of love are being planted each time Geri remembers to forgive herself and bring compassion to her sense of loss. Pausing helps her stop, appraise her situation more realistically, and recognize what is in her life now: good friends, fulfilling activities, and her own strengths that truly nourish and feed her.

· · · · · · · · · ·

STOP

What are your stressors? What do you believe about your ability to manage these stressors? What is the basis for these beliefs? How do they affect your actions?

· · · · · · · · · ·

Our beliefs are influenced by culture and our observation of others, especially people close to us. This subtle influence can be below the level of awareness but still affect our relationship to illness. My niece faints at the sight of a needle. Why? Her mother always faints when she has blood drawn or gets a vaccination. My niece had to learn that she could manage this task and didn't have to be afraid. The anticipatory anxiety exceeded the pain of an injection. Recently, she successfully completed a series of vaccinations she needed to work abroad. Her pride in mastering this fear will influence future events.

It is not always easy to know what we truly believe or why we do what we do. For example, I heard a story about a woman who cut off the end of a roast every time she cooked it. Her daughter asked her why she did this. The woman replied that her mother had done the same. Why had her mother cut off the end? It was because she didn't have a pot large enough to hold a whole roast.

. . . .

STOP

We are subject to conditioning and conditions. What are yours? Which ones would you like to cultivate further? Which ones need some weeding out?

. . . .

One afternoon, I was working on this chapter before a session with a patient. I closed my computer and told her what I was doing, adding, "Writing about stress is stressing me. It's such a big subject."

"Oh," she said. "You could write it about me."

"Really?" I said. "I haven't experienced you as particularly stressed. What are you experiencing that makes you say this?"

She stopped and thought. "Well, I worry all the time."

"All the time?" I asked. (This is an example of remembering the bad and forgetting all those times when worry is absent.) "What do you worry about?"

"Everything," she said.

I knew this was an exaggeration, but she believed it to be true. As we began to investigate this feeling, it became clear that some of her worries were appropriate and limited to specific situations, while others were more generalized and chronic. The cancer she had left her with some permanent impairment that was uncomfortable and continually reminded her that the cancer could return.

"What are you worried about right now?" I asked.

"My sixteen-year-old daughter is going sledding tonight," she said.

Her answer surprised me. I had expected her to say, "The return of my cancer." Her doctor had told her she was cured, but she was having a hard time believing it. Her reason for entering therapy was to stop worrying excessively and be better able to discern when she needed to be concerned. I was happy that she was concerned about her daughter's safety. This fear was current and realistic. As a parent, she needed more information. Where was her daughter going sledding? Was it in a dark area or on a well-lit hill that was safe and protected? Who was she going with, and how safety conscious were they? Answers to those questions could help my patient determine whether there was a real cause for concern and, if so, the appropriate action. Upon examination, she realized that her daughter was going with friends to a place she knew was safe. She felt reassured that her daughter could be trusted not to act foolishly. Unlike her worries over her health, she could resolve this stressor. Her faith in her daughter's judgment was reaffirmed, and she could let the worry go.

What do you fear? How realistic is it? Do you believe that you can put it in perspective and let it go?

Reflection

What causes you stress? You can explore this thought with a partner or write out your responses.

My stressors:

_____

_____

_____

_____

_____

My reaction (automatic):

_____

_____

_____

_____

_____

How I would like to respond:

_____

_____

_____

_____

_____

10 / Coping

Attitude is a little thing that makes a big difference.
—*Winston Churchill*

Some of my patients are in a support group, and they had been encouraging me to visit and lead them in a meditation. I know the leader of this group, a wonderful woman named Nina, and she welcomed my participation in a session. I think support groups are a wonderful way to connect with others who, like you, know what it is to face death and undergo treatment that is often debilitating. I have been meeting with my own group of women friends since we recovered from our stem cell transplants. (Women seem to be more apt to form a group than men.) They are an important part of my life and well-being, so I was looking forward to attending my patients' group.

When the day came, I arrived a little early to talk to Nina. As we were chatting, an alarm went off. We disregarded it at first and then learned that it was real: a woman from the group was having a seizure in the pool at the Y where we were meeting. Nina was called in, and the other group members waited nervously with me to see if the woman would be all right. Just that day she had e-mailed them, telling them that her doctor had discovered a brain tumor.

As I waited, I could feel a lump in my throat and a heaviness in my chest. This was not part of my plan for the meeting. Everyone stayed calm, but it was very disturbing. When the ambulance came, Nina went with the woman to the hospital, and I was left with the group. As latecomers straggled in, they were given the news.

In-breath. Out-breath.

My heart was beating rapidly. Watching the woman taken out on a stretcher with an oxygen mask on her face had brought back memories of my hospitalization. I had planned to talk about coping and adapting to change, and here it was, right in front of me. I needed a few moments to calm and center myself.

"Let's take a minute," I said, "and just settle."

We briefly quieted. Then Elizabeth, one of the women who had been in the pool at the time, took charge and said, "As you all know, Janet learned this morning that she has a brain tumor. She had a seizure by the pool, but she will be all right."

I admired Elizabeth's ability to speak clearly and with authority. She was my patient, and I felt proud of her calm and lucidity. Only later did I wonder if it had been an icy quiet that comes with shock.

Angela, her friend and my other patient, spoke next. She herself had been treated twice for brain tumors. "Janet has a strong faith in Jesus. He was with her today, because she got the right attention. Another person in the pool was a nurse who had experience with seizures and knew just what to do. Also, the lifeguard noticed something wasn't right, and he caught Janet, stopping her fall. It was a miracle."

I thought how wonderful that, in this time of crisis, Angela could focus on the power of faith. I knew how worried she was about her own health. As she spoke, I remembered the words of my oncologist: "The one thing that helps people the most through their illness is faith." Angela, who was not particularly religious, told me later that she interpreted faith as "anything that keeps you in touch with what makes you hopeful."

I paused after Angela and Elizabeth finished so we could absorb this information. Then as a group, we all closed our eyes; connected to the rhythm of breath moving through our bodies; and held Janet in our hearts and minds, sending her our caring thoughts and good wishes for health. As we sent her these thoughts of love and healing, I also recommended that we receive them ourselves.

"What helps you cope?" I asked the women in the group.

Four of the liveliest ones were in their eighties. One of them said, "I just push on."

"You certainly do," said her friend. "You had eight children."

We laughed, and I asked if this had been her major way of coping before cancer too.

"Yes," she said. "I had to."

Another woman said that she often quoted a passage from the Bible about strength. She couldn't remember it exactly but thought it was from Philippians: "I can do all things through Christ, who strengthens me" (Philippians 4:13).

A third said she found something each day that made her feel good. Another member confessed that she sang to herself from a repertoire of songs that she found inspirational.

Our experiences prior to being sick also affect our appraisal of our illness and how we cope. We may have watched someone close to us die and believe that our death will follow the same pattern. This is not likely to be true, but we may believe it anyway. No disease acts exactly the same in all people, and life experiences vary just as personalities and approaches do. It was interesting to note how each person in the group had her own unique style of coping. Elizabeth was a take-charge person and was accustomed to giving orders; Angela liked caring for others and was her family's peacemaker.

A patient of mine who had watched the painful death of her mother feared that she would suffer through the same prolonged agony. She didn't know that there have been leaps in palliative care and symptom control since her mother's death. The hospice workers I know wish people would call them in earlier. They feel that many suffer unnecessarily due to their reluctance to acknowledge that they are nearing death and that they and their families need help.

It is not always easy to be aware of the beliefs we hold and how they help or hinder us. I believe it is possible to have equanimity about cancer, but I can't believe I'll *never* be anxious or upset. Just the other day, I observed my anxiety as I sat waiting for the results of a mammogram. There were body memories of having been in radiology the year before and a mass in my breast being discovered. I felt my heart beating more quickly and noticed that my respiration was more shallow and my thoughts more rapid. This was conditioned reaction based on experience. No exam has been routine for me since I was first diagnosed with lymphoma in 1995. Each time, I prepare myself psychologically by acknowledging my nervousness. It is not useful (or possible) to block it. I tell a few people close to me when I am going for a checkup and ask that they send me their good wishes. I breathe, bring an interesting book, and tell myself, "I'll get through this."

· · · · · · · · · ·

I'll get through this. I can manage.

· · · · · · · · · ·

Even as I write now, I notice my hands growing a little sweaty. In my mind, there is a danger light blinking. It's automatic. I know I will cope with whatever happens, but I still hope that I won't have to move through another bout of cancer—I know that recurrences happen with my type of lymphoma. Reaching out to others, talking, and receiving their support helps me manage my anxiety.

In the waiting room that day, there were four other women, three of whom were in hospital gowns like me, also waiting. One woman, fully dressed, was bent over the thick notebook on her lap. She had an IV port in one arm.

"It hurts," she said, referring to the port.

We all looked up and learned that she had just been diagnosed. I could almost feel again what it was like at the beginning of chemotherapy. My veins had hurt also before I'd had a central line put in to administer the drugs directly.

Another woman, young and clearly anxious, now felt free to tell us she was there for a consult. She, too, had just received a diagnosis and was deciding whether it was worth traveling to this hospital and its doctors for treatment rather than going to one closer to her home. (We all told her, yes, it was worth it; she was in good hands.)

I confided that I was writing this book and asked the other women if there was anything helpful they would like to say to others. I promised I would include it. At first, there was silence, and then the woman sitting diagonally opposite from me said, "I do."

"Yes?"

"I lived in Morocco for a while," she said, "and there people pray five times a day."

"It's a tape," one of the other women said.

"Yes. You've been there?"

"I've traveled," was the response.

Now that the first woman had our attention, she went on to describe how she found it helpful to evoke a sense of a greater being and bring to mind an inspirational thought or scene. The practice brings peace and is inspirational, like the prayers in Morocco.

The woman who had traveled added, "I pause and acknowledge gratitude."

"For what?" I asked.

"I say to myself that I'm grateful I am not in pain, I'm grateful for my husband, I'm grateful for my friends, I'm grateful that I'm not afraid, I'm grateful that I am at peace."

We all listened, and I felt my spirit lift and the mood in the waiting room shift.

The young woman with the IV began to speak. "I have my notebook here," she said. "This helps me. I have a plan."

We looked at her. This was early in the game, and we all knew that anything could happen.

She went on to describe the course of her treatment, first this, then that. "It's all here," she said, lifting up her notebook. "I'm a teacher. I'm used to planning. This helps me. I also have a large family. I'm the ninth of ten children. I have a lot of support."

Discussion continued as I was called in to hear the results of my mammogram. This time, nothing was discovered. I breathed a sigh of relief and returned to the women in the waiting room, aware that their news might be different from mine. I was moved by the mutuality of support and caring expressed among us, all strangers but connected and wishing each other well. We were all doing our best to make sense of our disease and maintain our spirits.

One of my coping mechanisms is to seek out inspirational stories and hold them in my mind. Milton Erickson, a famous hypnotherapist whose work I have studied, is one of those stories. He had polio as a young man, which left him paralyzed. He tells the story of overhearing the doctors tell his parents one particularly grim day that he would be dead in the morning. He remembers growing intensely angry when he heard this. Sidney Rosen, in the book *My Voice Will Go with You*, transcribed what Erickson told him had happened immediately afterward:

> My mother then came in with as serene a face as can be. I asked her to arrange the dresser, push it up against the side of the bed at an angle. She did not understand why, she thought I was delirious. My speech was difficult. But at that angle by virtue of the mirror on the dresser I could see through the doorway, through the west window of the other room. I was damned if I would die without seeing one more sunset. If I had any skill in drawing, I could still sketch that sunset.

If it were true that he would be dead in the morning, he did not want to miss any moment of beauty. I admired this response. It's how I want to live my life.

"I used to think big," said a patient of mine who lives with lupus. "But now they're moments of rest, being outside, playing with my dog, seeing a beautiful moment, a warm breeze, feeling the rain. We are all vulnerable. Things can change in the blink of an eye. I appreciate the small things. Love and kindness make a difference. I like being helpful to others."

· · · · · · · · · ·

We are all connected. Love and kindness make a difference.
We are not alone.

· · · · · · · · · ·

STOP

What helps you cope?

· · · · · · · · · · ·

Choosing sayings that are inspirational and meaningful is helpful. After my dentist heard that I had lymphoma, I remember his telling me, "We only get what we are strong enough to bear." I didn't like that concept and didn't find it comforting. In contrast, my father had a sign hanging on his wall that said, "You cannot prevent the birds of sorrow from flying over your head, but you *can* prevent them from building nests in your hair." He also had a placard that said, "To get to the other side, you have to leave the shore." Those sayings fit me better. What are yours?

Music can be another wonderful way to lift the spirit and keep us going. On the wall in one of the transplant units at Dana Farber in Boston, the word *Believe* is written in bold blue letters. It is bright and cheerful and a wonderful contrast to the hospital environment. I liked it but had no idea what it meant. Later, I discovered it was from a song by Josh Groban from the movie *Polar Express:*

Believe in what your heart is saying,
Hear the melody that's playing.
There's no time to waste,
There so much to celebrate.
Believe in what you feel inside,
Give your dreams the wings to fly.
You have everything you need, if you just believe.

STOP

What gives you meaning? Are there any sayings or songs that inspire and enrich how you approach your illness?

· · · · · · · · · · ·

The coping strategies I have described here are primarily emotion-focused. At the pool, when the nurse sat by the woman who was having a seizure and knew how to care for her, that was problem-focused. We need both the emotional stamina to keep ourselves well and the ability to strategize and problem solve. Certain conditions support our well-being, while others do not.

A patient of mine who has heart disease and has been hospitalized several times for heart failure carries with her a photograph she took of a favorite place at the beach. It is a picture of waves crashing on the rocks, and on it, she has written the question "What could I do if I were not afraid?"

This is a woman who loves to be active. One of her great pleasures was skiing. She can no longer ski the expert slopes high on the mountain as she used to do, but she can still go to the mountain. She now sits in the lodge, enjoys the companionship of other skiers, and takes some runs on the lower and easier slopes. Her fears are valid and need attending, but she works at keeping them in perspective. She respects her limitations, listens carefully to the rhythm of her heart and her fatigue level, but does not let them keep her from everything she loves.

Another patient of mine is very visual. She creates art to express themes that are inspirational to her using words or phrases that evoke positive memories. She also does this for others based on what helps them feel good or is meaningful to them. It makes her happy to do these paintings, and she gives them away .

Reflection: My Coping Styles

What inspires you to live each moment and maintain curiosity and interest?

What beliefs support your ability to feel inner peace?

Do you believe that you have some control over your life, even when you are ill?

What are your coping strategies?

Do you refresh them daily?

I recommend finding a quiet place where you won't be interrupted and either listening to the audio (available for download at www .shambhala.com/BeingWell) and following one of the meditations or sitting silently and allowing the mind to quiet. When you feel settled, ask yourself the preceding questions. Let the answers emerge free of judgment or censure. You may do this more than once and observe what arises. Responses may vary. Feel free to jot them down.

Kindness and Compassion

To meet pain, accept pain, and bear pain, we need support, and we need to remember to be kind and compassionate to ourselves as well as to others. I believe that I am here today because many people sent me love and wishes to be well when I was ill. One of my teachers, Sharon Salzburg, who authored *Lovingkindness* and is one of the founders of the Insight Meditation Society, says it helps her to know that every day someone is sending her loving-kindness, or *metta*. A friend of mine who is a long-term meditator was coping quite well with a diagnosis of cancer until she developed an infection that was painful and life-threatening. She sent e-mails to friends and colleagues to help her get through this time. "I had to call in the troops," she says.

I was glad she had. Many of my patients have created websites to update friends and family about their condition and allow people to respond. One patient of mine told me how much it meant to her as she went through surgery. She was too weak to speak to anyone but could read the comments of people wishing her well.

Every day, as I complete my meditation, I take a moment to hold in my heart those in need, both people I know and others beyond my circle of friends. It is very comforting, and it helps me feel that I am doing something even when I am not able to be with a person physically.

A colleague of mine, Phyllis Pilgrim, spent a number of years of her childhood in a Japanese prison camp in Java. To survive and remain emotionally intact, her mother told her and her little brother to see something beautiful, say something beautiful, and do something beautiful every day. It could be sharing a piece of bread with another or letting an elder have a drink of water before they did, a smile, the sight of a flower growing in the dirt—something simple but hugely important to maintaining their spirits in terrible circumstances. Similarly, a monk in Burma who had been imprisoned for twenty-nine years remarkably was not angry, bitter, or defeated. When asked if he had been afraid during this time, he said, "Of only one thing—that I would lose my compassion." Thinking of another and caring for the hurt person(s) inside his captors helped him maintain his dignity and sense of worth.

Compassion can be defined as a quivering of the heart. My heart quivers when someone I love is sick. When someone dies prematurely—a child, a friend, a family member, or our dearly beloved—grief can make us question everything about living. We can respond with hatred or with love. There is a story about a mother wolf and her two cubs, one named Love and the other Hate. She has only enough food to feed one. Which one will survive? The answer is the one she feeds.

. . . .

STOP

What do you feed?

. . . .

My patient Ann has had a hard life, but a source of joy for her has been her daughter, Pam, who is her only living child. Pam needed some corrective surgery, and Ann volunteered to take her to the hospital and wait to take her home. Pam was sedated and taken to the operating room early, but an emergency delayed her surgery. As Ann anxiously waited for her daughter, she began talking to the other people in the waiting room. She later described to me how they formed a community of mutual support and comfort. Shortly after her daughter had finally gone into the operating room, Ann's son-in-law, waiting nervously at home, called her. She was in the midst of a conversation and inadvertently pressed the speaker on the phone.

"What the hell is going on?" he yelled, so loudly that he could be heard throughout the waiting room. "Why don't those bastards move on it? What's f—ing wrong with them?"

His blasphemy continued to broadcast, impossible to silence. Mortified, Ann quickly went into the corridor and explained to her son-in-law that surgery had been delayed but was currently in progress. Her calm shaken, she hung up as soon as she could and went back into the waiting room, where she apologized to everyone.

"He's just very concerned about his wife," she told them, embarrassed and disturbed.

After telling me this story, she paused and turned in her chair to look at me. "Life goes on, and you can choose which way to go," she said. "I focus on the kindness of people and the beauty that is present."

As we held the space of her disappointment that this man reminded her of her ex-husband, her daughter's father, who was alcoholic and abusive, the doorbell rang. Since my office is in my home, I excused myself in the midst of this tender moment, rushed downstairs, and realized it was the dog groomer. Chagrined that I hadn't been prepared for her and forestalled this interruption, I ran back upstairs to leash the dog, who did not want to go and had ignored my command to come. After I had taken her down to the groomer, I returned upstairs and took some breaths.

"I'm so sorry," I said.

Ann simply smiled and told me how the dog had hidden behind the chair when I went down to see who was at the door. "She knew," she said.

"It goes on, and you can choose which way to go," she repeated, telling me more about the day in the hospital. When her daughter was out of recovery and they were leaving the hospital, it was late and dark, and they were exhausted. My patient is in her seventies and has a heart condition. She also has trouble seeing in the dark, and it was sleeting and snowing. Home was a few hours away; soon they were caught in a two-hour gridlock in traffic, and her daughter's anesthesia was wearing off.

"I was very tired," Ann said. "I could have panicked, but I told myself that I had to keep calm, and I did. I look to the kindness that's present. I remembered the people in the hospital who were so caring, the fact that there was gas in the car and my daughter was there with me."

This patient has had many tragedies in her life: a son who overdosed as a young man in his twenties; another son, an alcoholic, who cannot be located; and an aging, infirm husband who had totaled their car the week before, two days before he was to have surgery.

"It goes on," she repeated. "Even the dog knew there was no escape. Might as well surrender and choose peace."

What sustains us? What can we connect to that allows us to let go, mourn, and continue in our lives without fear or ill will? Grief can force us to grow bigger and connect to the vastness of love and the spaciousness of peace. I have been most inspired by people like Ann. Rumi, the Persian poet of the thirteenth century, tells us we can never revert to what was before: bread cannot become wheat again, nor can a mirror turn back into iron. But even a change for the worse can mature us. Be secure, he says, and become the light.

Faith helps us find the light we seek, but it is also awareness that we are not alone that supports our efforts to be compassionate and kind. I recently told an acquaintance that I taught a course on kindness at the Center for Mindfulness, and he looked at me with a questioning expression.

"I wouldn't think anyone would need a course on that," he said.

Sadly, we do. Many people showed up to my class and helped each other practice kindness. They intentionally cultivated compassion and breathed with vulnerability, self-criticism, and forgiveness. They committed themselves to noticing their own strengths and to self-nourishing. Somehow, we seem to be so busy that we forget to care for ourselves wisely. We need to learn to remember that we cannot help another unless we are strong ourselves. I love to quote Rabbi Hillel,

If I am not for myself, who will be?
If I am only for myself, what am I?
If not now, when?*

In this society, it is often easier to bring compassion to others than to ourselves. Caregivers seem especially vulnerable to this lapse. Today, I came back from being with a group of hospice workers. Once a month, I go to their agency to lead the staff, social workers,

---

*Ethics of the Fathers 1:14.

Kindness and Compassion 101

nurses, administrators, and chaplain in meditation and provide a forum to talk. These people selflessly give of themselves daily without much support or acknowledgment. The agency is understaffed and underfunded, and each person is pressured to see a certain number of people each day. This once-a-month, ninety-minute meeting is their only time to be together and share the challenges, pains, and joys of their work with the dying. No other space is set aside for self-care and reflection. Their weekly staff meeting is problem-focused. The pain they carry is often silent, invisible, and unrecognized. As a result, many of the nurses feel they do not have the time to come to the meeting, and if they do, they often complain of being burned out.

Today, I began the session with a meditation and felt a sense of struggle and disquiet.

"I noticed a restlessness today," I said, after we ended. "I wonder if this reflects any of the frustration and stress you're experiencing at work."

Sadly, the answer was yes; they were feeling irritable and overwhelmed. There was too much to do and not enough time to do it. One of the social workers said, "Sometimes I am sitting with a patient, and I am thinking about productivity rather than being present to the person I'm with."

The chaplain, who is new to this agency, reported her disappointment that they didn't use their weekly staff meetings to reflect on the good things that had happened during the week rather than focusing only on problems. When she began work, she had been told to attend these weekly meetings but to keep her comments short. She was unable to hold the space or offer more than some brief inspirational readings that she selected.

Noting how few people had come to this meeting, which was specifically set aside as a time for reflection and support, I asked the group, "Is it a hardship for you to come here?"

"I went out of my way to be here this morning," Holly, one of the nurses, answered. "Mr. F. is dying." She teared up as she spoke.

"Yes, you've been with him a year and become very close to him. Every time he sees you, he smiles," said one of the social workers.

"I've tried not to get too emotional, but . . ." She could no longer speak through her tears.

"Tears are like baptism," said the chaplain. "They are tears of mercy. It helps not to be alone."

This reminded me of the figure of Christ on the cross that had been pinned to the wall of my room in the hospital when I was receiving chemotherapy. At the time, I didn't understand why it was there, and it reminded me of the tubes sticking into my body. I knew it was supposed to bring comfort, but instead it seemed to remind me of my own pain.

I mentioned this to the chaplain, and she told me that Christ was there to help us bear our own suffering so we would not feel alone. "I wish I had known that," I told her. "It would have been helpful." Jewish tradition teaches that the *shekhina,* God's intimate presence, dwells at the bedside of anyone who is ill.*

The nurses, the social workers, the chaplain, and all the others at this meeting act in this capacity. They create a presence of companionship and comfort, compassion they don't often receive themselves.

"Let's name all the people whom we have been with whom we'd like to remember and have not had a chance to grieve," I suggested.

Another person said, "Let's hold hands."

With care, we tightened our circle; joined hands; and slowly, from

---

* Babylonian Talmud, Tractate Nedarim 40a.

deep in our hearts, allowed the image and sense of those whom we have touched and who have touched us to be named.

Peace.

A Guided Meditation on Love and Kindness

This meditation is designed to cultivate a sense of love and kindness. The phrases listed here are the ones that I repeat to myself on a regular basis. I do them as a formal practice, and I keep them in my heart and head to use informally when I need an extra boost of kindness and understanding, either toward another or toward myself. The meaning of the words is more important than the words themselves. As you say the phrases to yourself, find the ones that truly resonate with you. The words are changeable, but the intention to foster a state that cultivates love and kindness is timeless.

This meditation is like cultivating a garden. You may notice weeds among the growing flowers. These are negative mind states like anger, self-pity, resentment, and frustration. Sadness also can arise. This is normal, and if you allow these states to come, they will fall away. Gardens do not grow overnight. We cannot force them into being; water them with patience and understanding, and watch how they grow.

A Loving-Kindness Meditation

May I be safe and protected (free from danger).
May I be happy (in body and mind).
May I be healthy (in mind and body, resilient and strong).
May I live with ease (peace and contentment).

Instructions for Meditation

1. Begin in a comfortable position. Adjust the temperature in the room or have a blanket nearby to warm you should you feel cool.

2. Let your eyes close and bring to mind an image or feel a sense of a person who has been good to you and whom you love and appreciate. Hold this person in your heart, embracing his love and kindness and sending it forth. Say each of the preceding phrases, or focus on words of your choosing, and direct these wishes to this person. Repeat the phrases and continue directing their meaning to this person as long as you like.

3. When you feel ready and have established stability of attention and a sense of connection to the meaning of each phrase, you may expand these wishes to yourself.

4. Feel free to adjust the phrases so that you can really connect to their meaning. Repeat each one to yourself as often as you like, moving from one phrase to another as you are ready, again and again. There is no time limit.

5. When you have a sense of fullness, you can move on to a neutral person and send these wishes to someone for whom you have no special feelings, perhaps a clerk in a store or a casual acquaintance.

6. When you are ready, you can expand these wishes and send them to a person (or even a part of yourself) with whom you have difficulty. Do not be concerned if you do not immediately feel any effect from this meditation. You will be practicing a more spacious and loving attitude toward yourself and others. In time, you may notice an increased sense of compassion, wisdom, and well-being as well as happiness about the happiness of others.

7. You may continue expanding the circle to whom you send these wishes, including all sentient beings and even inanimate objects. Do this gently and lovingly, with tenderness, as often as you like.

12 / Thoughts on Thinking

The world we have created is a product of our thinking; it cannot be changed without changing our thinking.

—*Albert Einstein*

You cannot plough a field by turning it over in your mind.

—*Anonymous*

A student sitting with his teacher one day was having difficulty concentrating on his lesson. The bank where they were sitting was high, and below was a raging river filled with rocks. He could not stop himself from looking at the wild river below him and worrying that he would slip off the bank and fall into it. Finally, not able to contain his fear, he spoke. "Tell me, teacher. Am I in danger of falling in the river and drowning?" he asked.

"No," said the teacher. "It isn't falling in that causes you to drown; it's staying in."

How often do we worry about a future that may never happen instead of the ground beneath our feet? It is easy to get lost in a round of negative thoughts that are frightening and disabling. Cancer, chemotherapy, radiation, and strong medications assault the whole system. As the body fights what is wrong, it is often difficult to experience what is right. It is normal to struggle with a variety of feelings.

Sometimes we cannot maintain a loving, positive attitude, but that doesn't mean we are failures or are hastening our death.

Patients come to me upset because they are upset and cannot get out of their own way. John, a prominent therapist, was one such patient. Normally confident and upbeat, he was referred to me by his doctor because he was tormenting himself with repetitive thoughts. Even though John had successfully completed treatment for his lymphoma and was feeling fine physically, his mind could not stop creating catastrophes. Thoughts of being ill, dying, and experiencing pain kept popping into his head. These thoughts were repetitive and intrusive. He could not push them away or stop them. Every twinge in his body activated fear of a recurrence or a second cancer that would destroy his body, create intolerable pain, and end his life. He was angry and upset that he couldn't control these thoughts or free himself from them. In his mind, he knew that he was catastrophizing, but this knowledge only increased his self-disgust and fear.

John sat in my sunlit office, talking animatedly and nonstop about his distress. He was blind to the sight of the evergreen trees visible through the window, the beauty of the day, and the comfort of his chair. He was very analytical and insightful, aware that he was intensifying his distress and creating his own torture. "But I can't stop it," he said angrily. "I think about cancer all the time. I'm driving my family—and myself—crazy. They can't understand it."

I listened, nodding my head numerous times and agreeing that these feelings were disturbing. I didn't try to reassure him or show him the falsity of his views. A whole chorus of people—his wife, his friends, and even his children—had been trying to convince him that everything was fine. Their efforts, though well meaning, were only making him feel worse. I knew that anything I said would intensify his distress and cause more resistance.

As John talked, I observed how hard he was trying to "keep it all together" and how harshly he was judging himself. When I noticed his speech speeding up and his agitation escalating, I asked him if he would be willing to stop, take a moment, and go inside to notice how his body was reacting. He was willing to try, so he leaned back in the recliner in my office, closed his eyes, and felt his breath.

He noted a tightening in his belly, constriction in his throat, and discomfort in his chest. Gently, I asked him to place his hand on his belly and feel how breath was moving the belly. "Imagine it's like a balloon, inflating with air and deflating," I told him. "Don't try to change anything; just let yourself feel its movement."

After he did this for a minute or two, I had him open his eyes and instructed him to look out the window and notice what met his gaze. He did so in silence, and after a minute or two, I asked him, if he were willing, to return to his breath and focus on it again. He could do so with his eyes open or closed.

"Thoughts will pop in," I told him. "Don't try to push them away. Note them and continue bringing your attention back to your breath. You can also check into your body and experience how it feels as you catch yourself thinking."

I sat there quietly while he did this, also noting how my own body felt and the rhythm of my breath. I hoped that this process of noting, allowing, and investigating the effect of thought (and the emotion that went with it) would be freeing for him.

This process took about ten minutes, but during that time, his attention shifted. For this brief period, his mind was occupied with sensation, the feeling of his hand resting on his belly, the movement of the belly, the feel of breath, and the challenge of catching thought and redirecting attention to breath and body. Even his harsh judging could be observed with greater neutrality. Shifting attention (not trying to stop the thought but to feel the breath) created some space between him and his thoughts.

"How wonderful," I said. "Each time you notice yourself caught up in a chain of thoughts, note 'thinking,' and bring your attention back to your direct experience—be it auditory, visual, or kinesthetic—you are developing your mindfulness muscle."

By looking outside himself and through the window, John temporarily filled his mind with a different scene, and it was based on his direct experience as it was unfolding rather than on an imaginary scenario. This helped him to identify less with fear, shame, and the thoughts that he was "bad" or a failure.

"You know your thoughts are conditioned," I told him. "You can even be curious about them, when they come, when they go. You can even label the thought. Call it 'worry,' 'planning,' 'problem solving,' 'doubting,' 'judging,' whatever it might be. If there is a feeling, an emotion, you can name it too. You can even say to yourself, 'Hating, hating.' Let yourself be curious. You can experiment with this process and see what happens. These thoughts and feelings are normal. How wonderful that you can allow them to emerge. They're just thoughts, like feathers in the wind."

John left my office, and I didn't hear from him again. I had no idea whether he had followed my suggestions. A year or two later, I saw him at a conference. He came up to me and said, "Thank you, you really helped me."

Puzzled, because I remembered wondering whether the session with me had been useful, I asked, "How did I help?"

"You helped me realize my feelings were normal," he said. "You gave me permission to be upset. This helped me to stop judging myself so harshly. After a while, I could say to myself, 'Thinking.' I take a breath, and it grounds me. I'm less at the mercy of my thoughts. Sometimes when I find myself absorbed by worry or negative feelings, I look out the window or at a friendly face."

He smiled as he spoke. It was clear he felt more in control and confident.

Permission to be upset, when you *are* upset, allows feelings to flow freely in and out, like breath. Their presence cannot be denied or forced away. *They must be acknowledged and met with compassion.* It is impossible not to be upset at times. The question is, how long does it last, and how quickly can you come back to a state of balance?

The breath or any other neutral object that is present and concrete can act as a life jacket, helping us stay afloat by shifting attention and expanding perspective. This takes practice. Please *don't* try to talk yourself out of thinking; rather, *allow, be curious, and continue strengthening your mindfulness muscle.* Be patient and persevere. The more quickly you can catch the thought and interrupt its pathway, the more you will see how transitory it is. A thought can be like putting a gun to your head. You can drop the gun by acknowledging the thought, feeling its effect, and observing what happens next. Instead of castigating yourself for thinking negatively, let it in and examine it. How wonderful: you have caught the thought rather than being caught in it. Now you can gently feel your breath and rope it in— much better than being critical of yourself for having it. Thoughts pass if we are willing to observe rather than react. Then we can ask ourselves, "How realistic is my thinking? What's the evidence?"

John knew that focusing on fear and worry was disabling, but he was powerless to prevent these feelings from arising; they were too ingrained. He needed permission to accept them before they could leave him. The ability to notice, accept, and refocus attention is cultivated. Like a child trying to walk, it takes a willingness to fall down and pick yourself up again until it is learned. Your intention to ride the current of thought and pull yourself out of the river and onto the shore is powerful. Thoughts can be like riptides; if you try to fight them, you will drown. Instead, you go with the current and swim parallel to the beach, even as the current carries you farther away. You will reach the edge of the riptide and then be able to swim out of it to the shore.

Being human, we will always be subject to times of discouragement, doubt, and fear. Anger will arise, as will irritability, frustration, restlessness, boredom, and fatigue. All of this is normal. These feelings are natural obstacles that the mind is subject to experiencing regardless of illness. Each is appropriate at different times, but often we allow them to define who we are rather than experiencing them as thoughts that are as ephemeral as a puff of smoke. They usually represent some kind of aversion to what is happening. This resistance to what cannot be changed is the gun that needs to be dropped. Treat your thoughts with respect; you need them, but note which ones help and which ones hinder your well-being.

Talking to yourself can be useful in countering negativity and maintaining perspective. Speak to yourself with affection, as if you were a small child who needed reassurance; treat yourself with love and concern. You need comfort and safety before you can hear reason. Ever try to reason yourself to sleep? Instead, you need to find something soothing and reassuring. It can be a glass of warm milk, a voice on a CD, a good book, soothing music, a calming presence, even a bubble bath. Whatever you like is much more effective than a stern lecture. Sometimes nothing works, and it's better to get up and occupy the mind with an activity rather than lying in bed and tossing and turning because you're too agitated to sleep.

When I was in the hospital and lying in bed, too weak to talk, I had my husband read me children's books. I loved *Little Toot*, which was about a small tugboat who isn't afraid to be a bit naughty and have fun riding the waves in the big, wild sea, a talent that makes him a hero later in the story. It brought back happy memories, and I could imagine myself being playful and free. I also liked to hear, "I think I can, I think I can," from *The Little Engine That Could*. It brought back good memories and was encouraging. I also liked inspirational stories that helped me believe in my own strength and resiliency.

Some conditions are more conducive to constructive thinking than others. A beautiful, sunny day can lighten a mood and create positive feelings. If the weather is dark and gloomy, we may need a reminder that this, too, shall pass. In some of my classes, I have had people create their own slogans to help them through difficult times. I have them write down words or phrases on index cards that help them maintain perspective. Some are Biblical sayings; others might be jingles from advertisements or maybe just a word or a memory. I have also asked people to illustrate their card or use an image instead of words. They can take the card and post it where it is visible. Most important, however, is to carry the thought in the heart as well as the head and be able to refer to it as needed. Thoughts are powerful. They can delight or frighten, but they never need to stay.

Meditation: Awareness of Thought

When your attention has become steady and your breath rhythmic and slow for a period of time, allow yourself to focus on thought. Notice when it arises and follow its path, as well as the spaces between one thought and another. If judging arises, observe judging; don't try to change anything or stop a thought. Follow its journey and connection to another thought. Notice if any patterns or repetitive thoughts emerge. Do sensations arise in the body? Do you comment on these sensations? Is there any leaning toward or away from certain thoughts? Are they pleasant or unpleasant? What is your relationship to what arises? If you find yourself drowning in thinking, lost in the thought, and being the thought mentally (being absorbed in the thought rather than witnessing it), come back to your breath as an anchor of attention. Do this for a set time. When you have finished, feel free to write down what you have learned.

. . . .

Letting be—letting go.

. . . .

Life is filled with surprises, especially if we are committed to living it fully. This can be both good and bad, but it is rarely what we expect. When I was younger, it was impossible to imagine myself having gray hair or looking like my mother. Possibilities seemed limitless and death far away. I took my body for granted, never conceiving of how it might change over time or that I would one day need to prioritize tasks and husband my energy to do what I once did with ease. Now I am happy that I am well enough to think about aging and how best to live each day. Focusing on my breath as an object of attention helps me experience both consistency and change, but even as I experience breath flowing in and out of my body, it is still shocking to know its nature is impermanent and that I will die.

Yesterday, Colleen, one of my patients, was driven to my office by her husband, John. A few days ago, she had a seizure. This meant her brain tumor was growing again, and the cancer was metastasizing more virulently. I did not want to hear this news. Immediately, as she sat down and began describing the event, my stomach began tightening, and I felt a constriction in my throat. As Colleen began crying, my eyes also filled with tears.

"I'm not ready to go," she said.

My body reacted right away. The lump in my throat grew, and I began coughing. My first thought was, "Oh, no. I'm not ready to have her go either." I knew I would adapt to this news, but now it was too fresh to accept. Yet I really wanted to be with her in her grief without being so consumed by it that I couldn't be helpful to her. Colleen identifies with her role as a mother, and I knew if I were not careful, she would be the one reassuring me instead of vice versa.

She was very concerned about upsetting her family, but at the same time, she recognized that she needed to be cared for herself. Knowing that she could no longer be the protector and go-to person for her loved ones intensified her grief.

"I wanted to grow old with John," she said, speaking of her husband. "When I had my seizure, I couldn't call for him, but I thumped on the chest in the bedroom where I was. He froze. He asked me what he should do. I couldn't talk, but I could move. I tapped 9-1-1 into the phone myself."

This was hard for me to hear. I could imagine how scared her husband must have been.

"He's my soul mate," she said. "My daughter came, but she was terrible."

"Terrible?" I was surprised because she had described her daughter as a take-charge person.

Colleen went on, "She told me, 'Mom, it's all about you.' She was very cold. I couldn't reason with her. She couldn't hear me. Finally, I just took her hands and told her it would be all right." She paused reflectively and added, "Her friend Sue will mother her. They're close. They talk."

I could feel the sadness, hers and mine. It seemed acceptance was intermingled with resignation, and as I listened to her, the realness and inevitability of death could not be denied. It was a reminder to me of how precious each moment is and how important it is to live it wisely. My own concerns seemed insignificant, and I hoped my husband and I would be able to go through retirement together and walk hand in hand as Colleen had envisioned doing with her husband.

We began talking a bit about decisions she would have to make. It was premature to think about the choices that might be available to her. Right now, we needed to focus on how she would get through the afternoon. It would be the first time she would be alone since the seizure, and she was scared.

"I'll keep busy," she said. "I've begun writing a love letter to John, and I'll do my taxes."

The session ended, and I helped her out, being careful to keep the dog away so she wouldn't trip. She was a bit shaky.

"You've taught me to live in the now," she told me. "It helps."

Yes, residing in the present does help, but it doesn't take away sadness, loss, and change. Only through acceptance of *this moment* and what it brings can we focus on what is possible. As long as we are alive, every breath is a reminder of the impossibility of holding on to what is gone. We can't stop change. We have to let go. We have no choice if we desire peace. Time and again as I listen to patients (and myself), I experience the misery of trying to grasp what cannot be contained. It's like holding water in the palm of your hand. It doesn't last, but you know it's been there.

As we made our way outside, Colleen expressed sorrow that she was upsetting people. She didn't want to cause pain, and it hurt her to see how others were affected by her illness. I acknowledged that I, too, was upset with her news.

"I'm sorry," Colleen told me.

"I'm not," I said. "How sad it would be if I didn't care."

"My husband said something similar about you. 'She loves you. We all do,' he told me."

It was a bright, sunny day that held the promise of spring, and Colleen wanted to sit on the lawn and wait there for her husband. I got a blanket to keep her warm and wrapped her up in it. It helped me to feel I was doing something to help, even as I knew this was just the beginning of a new journey that would lead to many good-byes and many changes, none of which were welcome.

How beautifully poet Mary Oliver expressed this moment in her poem "In Blackwater Woods":

To live in this world you must be able to do three things:
to love what is mortal;
to hold it
against your bones knowing your own life depends on it;

and, when the time comes to let it go,
to let it go.

Yesterday, Colleen was holding what she loved: some sunlight and her concern for others who were concerned for her. Letting be is not only accepting that death is approaching; it is also accepting the full range of thoughts, feelings, and sensations that arise.

It can hurt to love and to open your heart to a beloved who is hurting. Be you patient or caregiver, friend or acquaintance, it is human to want to hold on to what is dear and not let go. Everyone reacts differently to pain. It takes understanding and compassion to remember that this, too, changes—if we are willing to let it be and let go. Then love can enter and, with it, peace within the storm of change.

Meditation

Let yourself come into a position that best supports your body and mind. If you are sitting, feel the erectness of your spine and the alignment of your head with your body. If you are lying down, do so in a way that will help you to be comfortable and awake. Allow yourself to come to a place of rest by focusing on your breath or an object of attention that brings you to a state of peace. When your mind feels settled, you can let your eyes close (if they have not already) and bring attention into the area of your heart. Let yourself imagine this region surrounded by light and each heartbeat radiating through you, illuminating and warming each area of the body and lingering in areas of sensitivity and tenderness. Within this sphere of light, allow yourself to grieve what is gone.

13 / Decisions

"Sir, what is the secret of your success?"
a reporter asked a bank president.
"Two words."
"And, sir, what are they?"
"Good decisions."
"And how do you make good decisions?"
"One word."
"And sir, what is that?"
"Experience."
"And how do you get experience?"
"Two words."
"And, sir, what are they?"
"Bad decisions."

   —*Anonymous*

   In every moment of our lives, whether we realize it or not, it makes a difference where we place our attention. We are always making choices; some are conscious, while others seem to happen by circumstance or neglect and catch us by surprise. A series of decisions leads to every moment. Some are intuitive, and others come after much deliberation. Mindfulness-based stress reduction helps us connect to the heart, the head, and the body moment by moment. Being aware of the workings of our heart and mind as they unfold empowers us to make wiser decisions. We are able to notice our patterns of thought and the effect they have on our well-being. By observing with acceptance, we learn what contributes to health and what compromises it.

Many people come to me for assistance in decision making or to reconcile themselves to decisions that have resulted in negative consequences. It is difficult to predict the consequences of our actions in advance, especially if we are confronted with choices that could mean an extended life or death. I find that regret, self-blame, and recriminations need to be dropped to clearly assess priorities and evaluate what course is best. This requires a willingness to see clearly and know our inner selves. The more at rest the mind is when this happens, the greater our ability to sift through information, much of which can be contradictory and confusing.

When we are ill, there are different stages of decisions to make. The first is deciding to take control of what is possible, which is our attitude. Empowering ourselves to trust our inner wisdom allows us to act from our inner strength. For this, we need the courage to face what is true. This requires letting go of how we think our life should be and opening to it as it is. We must be willing to pay attention to the body and the mind with acceptance and define ourselves not by our illness but by our intrinsic worth.

A physician recently told me about a patient of his who had a phobia against doctors. Other than emergency surgery for a broken hip, she hadn't seen one in fifteen years. Her husband, also his patient, was very concerned and didn't know what to do to help her. She was losing weight, had weakness in one arm and difficulty walking, and was not eating well. During the husband's physical, he asked the doctor to call his wife. When he called and she realized it was the physician, she hung up on him. This, too, is a choice.

It is not always easy to confront the truth, but fear can be more harmful than whatever we fear. People worry about a cornucopia of symptoms; some may be normal, while others need attention. It takes discernment to know the difference and maintain perspective. I usually recommend that my patients see the doctor to check out a symptom and then let the worry go after they learn that all is fine— without judging themselves for a "false alarm." We may need to do this many times before we can truly be reassured that we are well.

Karen, a patient of mine who has stage IV breast cancer, discovered a swollen lymph gland under her arm. In the past, this symptom had signaled cancer. It frightened her, so she immediately called her physician, who examined it. Karen has a cat that had recently scratched her. Told that the swelling was probably an inflammatory response, she was given antibiotics and told to wait a week to see if it went down. She was still highly anxious when she saw me but determined to manage her anxiety. We discussed coping strategies: keep busy, continue doing yoga, see friends, and listen to guided meditations. She asked me if she could practice "softening into" her pain, so we spent some time meeting sensation (without labeling it "pain") without resisting it. This helped, but it didn't decrease her worries. It was realistic to be concerned, but I asked whether she could put this anxiety to rest before she went to sleep.

"Will worry change anything?"

"No," she admitted.

Fortunately, Karen was OK and it was an infection, but anxiety can be a signal that something is wrong. If it is overwhelming, it will cloud your judgment and create suffering. The sooner you recognize anxiety and the more you are able to STOP as soon as you feel yourself becoming anxious, the easier it becomes to refocus and center. Doing so with compassion rather than critical judgment gives you space and time to calm and gain a new perspective.

. . . .

STOP

What is in your awareness as you read this chapter? Allow your mind to quiet, and when it is settled, invite any worries you have about your physical health to enter into your awareness. Note the thought(s) and the sensations in the body that are present. How are you relating to these concerns? What evidence do you have about their significance? How realistic is your evidence? If fear is present, can it be held with compassion and understanding? What is your action plan? What is your coping strategy? What would letting it go feel like? Can you imagine it?

. . . .

The more we listen to the body, the more sensitive we become to its messages. A friend of mine, another teacher of mindfulness, has been a meditator for many years. She is deeply connected to her body and the workings of her mind. A number of years ago, she had a dream that indicated something was wrong with her breast. She had had a recent mammogram, and there was no evidence that anything was wrong. She didn't feel any lumps, and there was no family history of breast cancer. My friend, however, had learned to trust her intuition, so when the dream recurred, she had another mammogram. Breast cancer was discovered, and it was treated. Afterward, there were new decisions to make. To prevent recurrence, should she take the drug her doctor recommended or have more surgery? Was doing nothing a safe option? There were no guarantees, whatever she decided. Her task was to get as much information as possible, sift through it with a quiet mind, and ask herself how she would feel with the possible outcomes. Could she accept her decision and move on with a mind at rest, regardless of what might or might not occur?

Such decisions are difficult to make. There are often conflicting opinions and evidence. You and your family members may not agree on the same course of action—or inaction. We tend to want to "do something," but *something* can include choosing to do nothing: no additional procedures, treatments, or frequent tests. This is a valid option. When is enough, enough? What is our quality of life? How will it be affected by what we do? What about longevity? What are the odds that our lives will be prolonged? What are the potential costs and gains?

One woman in my practice decided that she did not want any more chemotherapy. She was fatigued and having many noxious side effects from it. She was very religious and accepting of her fate. She believed her time had come to die, but she wanted to be present for her daughter's wedding. She did everything possible to be here through that time and then elected to end treatment. Her family, her support group, and her husband were not happy with this decision. It was a difficult one, but as they saw her suffer not from cancer but from the side effects of treatment, they respected her wishes. She was able to die at home and at peace. Her tranquillity and acceptance of death eased their pain at her loss.

Another person who also had metastatic cancer came to see me when her condition worsened. This was her third bout with cancer, and she was on a maintenance dose of chemotherapy and had had a brain tumor removed a year before. She had a strong will to live and was determined not to "give up hope." Recently, her speech had become slurred, and she had some dizziness. After she experienced a seizure, she needed to decide whether to have more surgery to see what was causing her new symptoms. My patient sought the advice of three different doctors and had a CT scan, PET scan, and MRI to get as much information as possible. She and her family assessed risks and benefits, and only when her physician assured her that her functions would not be compromised did she decide to go ahead with the surgery. When a resident came to prepare her, she asked some last questions that he could not answer, so she refused the surgery that day. After her doctors consulted with each other, they came to talk with her, explaining that the tumor was too large to remove completely; their plan was to relieve some of the pressure in her brain. She then decided the surgery was worth the risk and chose to go ahead with it.

Decisions do not occur only on the physical level. When we were at our accountant's at tax time, we discussed the fact that my husband was thinking of retiring. We were concerned about our finances, a major worry when illness strikes. The accountant told us about his mother-in-law who, after her husband died, made a bucket list of things she wanted to do. After she died, he and his wife found this list in her wallet. Only a few items were checked off.

I don't personally feel I need to do anything extraordinary before I go, but I do not want to delay doing what I believe is important. I also treasure being able to talk and think and am not sure I would want to prolong treatment if my mind were going, and I could no longer communicate and needed life support to breathe. My awareness of the suddenness of change and the inevitability of death informs how I am living. This can range from marking an event and celebrating both small and large achievements to taking some extra time to be with a person who is close to me. I used to put things off and tell myself that I could do them later. I realize that the time is now, and there might never be a later time. For me, this is especially true in the area of relationships.

Since 1997, I have been meeting with a group of women who, like me, have had stem cell transplants. There are five of us. Initially, there were six, but one of the women died during the first year after our transplants. We meet about every six weeks, sometimes more often, other times less, but our friendship has continued throughout the years. We are not a traditional support group and rarely talk about cancer. Sometimes, we discuss the merits of repeated testing and the pros and cons of different treatments or health tips, but usually we talk about our families and daily activities. Some of us have had recurrences or more than one type of cancer, and others have not had a return of cancer since the stem cell transplant, but we are all well and share an appreciation of life and its gifts. None of us takes it for granted or puts anything off. At our last meeting, I asked them how cancer influenced the decisions they made.

Two of my friends immediately said, "Not at all."

Memories came back to my third friend and the first time she was diagnosed with cancer. Her children had been young. "It's different at different ages," she said. "Make sure you say that. When I was first diagnosed, the children were young, and I am the primary breadwinner. There were many implications, financial and otherwise. My husband made very little money, and I worried I wouldn't be able to raise my son and see him through school."

We all nodded. We're all older now, and most have adult children and grandchildren. I am the only one who's childless, but I, too, treasure family. I know how painful it is to be young and perhaps never have children because of chemotherapy or surgery. I also have cried with parents of young children who feel sad and sometimes guilty because they won't be there to guide their children and help them reach maturity. It is heartbreaking. I also know parents whose children have cancer, and they must face that stress and pain.

I was ready to change the subject when my fourth friend said, "Wait. You haven't heard from me."

This was said with a great deal of heat. She, too, had been young with a young family at her first diagnosis, and her children were still in elementary school when the cancer metastasized for the second time. The third time was two years ago, when a new cancer that was life-threatening and required major surgery was discovered. We were all worried about her survival. After she recovered, she decided to quit her job.

"I was a nurse," she recalled, "and I knew I couldn't be very sympathetic when a person came in with some minor complaint. I was working part-time but decided to quit. I decided to spend more time doing what I loved. Now I am no longer bothered by the small stuff.

"I'm now becoming a potter. When I was working in the studio and the kiln broke, another potter blamed me. It wasn't my fault, but I listened to her, decided it wasn't worth a battle, and apologized. People were surprised, but it wasn't important."

She paused. "Also, when I was going through it the third time, I didn't feel so good. It wasn't easy."

Heaviness descended over the table. We all have had cancer more than once. Now we are all thriving and busily engaged in activities, but this could cease at any time. We changed the topic.

In my experience, the will to live is very strong, regardless of age. No one wants to die prematurely; even at ninety-eight, it can feel too soon. I am not sure that the maxim "How we live is how we die" is wholly true, but I do know that how we live makes a difference not only to ourselves but also to all the people around us. Being concerned about loved ones of any age is normal. To write about illness is really to write about life and the quality of life.

Being at rest and at peace is a work in progress. It takes effort and honesty. After I recovered, I decided I didn't want to hold on to any knots I could still untie. As in Alcoholics Anonymous, I went back and made peace with some difficult people, asking forgiveness and forgiving. I do my best not to create new relationships filled with enmity and hurt. This intention helps me pause and take some breaths before I respond in anger. I can't always succeed, but I do my best not to cause harm or perpetuate injustice. Anger can be useful. It is energy, but it needs to be channeled skillfully. My intention to do no harm makes me consider my reactions and speech. I have had the good fortune to resolve some old hurts to others and myself. Ah. What a release to forgive—not to forget or give approval, but to drop what weighs on my heart and be free.

· · · · · · · · · ·

STOP

What is your aspiration for yourself? What allows you to feel whole and at peace? Are there any residues of enmity or hurt that you wish to resolve or release?

What is unfinished? How can you make peace with it? Remember, this is a process, and intention makes a difference and is powerful.

· · · · · · · · · ·

14 / Loss and Grief

The true condition of mind is like the sky, like space: without center, without edge, without goal.

   —*Shabkhar Rinpoche*

Birdwings

Your grief for what you've lost
lifts a mirror up
to where you're bravely working.
Expecting the worst,
you look
and instead,
here's the joyful face you've been wanting to see.
Your hand opens and closes
and opens and closes.
If it were always a fist
or always stretched open,
you would be paralyzed.
Your deepest presence
is in every small contracting and expanding,
the two
as beautifully balanced and coordinated
as birdwings.

   —*Rumi*

When we are ill, the rhythms of life take on a new cadence. Harmonizing with this rhythm may require letting go of preconceived ideas about how we think we should be and an acceptance of how we are. The body knows what it wants and needs, and if we listen and follow its lead, the mind will naturally come to a state of rest. With quiet and stillness, we can connect to a sense of spaciousness that enlarges our perspective and creates equanimity. Depending on our belief system, we may sense God or experience love. There is no striving to create this feeling. It comes from truly letting go. Within this space, difficult feelings and strong emotions can pass like clouds moving through the sky.

In the silence and stillness of meditation, feelings we might have buried or tried to push away are able to emerge. As we recognize loss and open to sorrow, tears can flow, and we may have crying spells. This is a healing part of the grieving process, but because it is uncomfortable, we may resist its emergence. We may feel weak if we cry. We may worry about the effect of our tears on others. We may be embarrassed and apologetic for exposing our vulnerability. This hesitation interrupts the flow of connection and imprisons us in our own suffering. A touch, a smile, a caring presence soothes the pain of loss and is beneficial. Our hearts can break open yet receive support.

Our reluctance to display our grief may be cultural and arise from how we think we should be rather than how we are. There is nothing to be ashamed of when we cry or display grief. It happens. It is not bad or good. It is human.

May our hearts break open rather than close.
May we open to love and compassion.

Loss is inevitable, but it can be accelerated by serious illness.

Some losses are huge, while others are subtle. There can be a slow diminution of function or a sudden, life-altering change. A few days before she was to leave the country to complete her education, a young woman discovered she had a sarcoma that was very serious. She needed immediate treatment, which interrupted all her plans. She was nearing completion of a graduate program and in a new serious relationship. She was ready to embark on a rich career and an equally satisfying life when she learned she did not have long to live. Refusing to die before her time, she entered therapy to suppress her symptoms, went on her trip, and completed her degree. She is now continuing to manage her disease and preparing to work, rock climb, and enjoy everything she can while she can. Her family is grieving, as are the young woman and her lover, but she is fully alive for now.

Physiological changes create limitations, decreasing mobility and diminishing functionality. What we once took for granted is now an effort. Our lives change. We may have to stop working, which creates financial hardships as well as a loss of identity. Time is compressed, and with it comes a contraction of possibilities; what you thought you could do "tomorrow" may never be achieved.

It is not easy to move from independence to greater dependence and the need to rely on others. We may drown in regret, clinging to the past and being miserable in the present. None of this is abnormal or even destructive as long as it is temporary. Being well when we are sick does not mean we are immune to grief. Wellness does not mean never getting angry, feeling sad, or having feelings that are disturbing and painful. Elisabeth Kübler-Ross, a psychiatrist and pioneer in near-death studies, described five stages of grief: denial, anger, bargaining, depression, and hope or acceptance. We experience all of these stages but not necessarily in a specific order. There is no right way to grieve and no timescale for reaching acceptance. Much depends on culture and personality.

My father had diabetes and heart disease in his later years, preventing him from fully partaking in his lifelong joy and satisfaction: food. No more visits to the deli for a good pastrami sandwich or salami hanging on the hinge of the door, readily available to eat. When he learned he also had cancer, he had to leave the town where he was born and the friends he'd known from childhood to live with us. During this process of change, he would say, "Getting old isn't for sissies."

I'd laugh when he said it, but when I later became ill and felt older than my age, I understood. The energy that had enabled me to have a private practice in psychotherapy, train professionals in stress reduction, teach MBSR, and be socially active fizzled. I lost my identity as I became the one needing services rather than the caregiver. When I could return to work, I was different emotionally and physiologically. Certain opportunities were lost. My energy had lessened, and I had to consider how to pace myself throughout the day. I needed time to recover and renew. I had to learn to say "No." I had to remember that I couldn't do all that I wanted when I wanted it. When I decided it was worth expending energy beyond my comfort zone, I had to accept the consequences of fatigue.

Illness and loss affect everyone in our circle, especially those to whom we are close. Henrietta, a patient of mine who lives with congestive heart failure, has been hiding the seriousness of her condition from her daughter. She fears upsetting her. Recently, she and her daughter went to an exceptionally beautiful horticultural garden. They had lunch, and afterward her daughter took her for a walk along a loop in the meadow. It was a beautiful spring day filled with the glory of budding trees and fresh blooming flowers, but the path was uphill, and Henrietta had to go very slowly. She had to pause every few steps to catch her breath. Her daughter, seeing how labored her mother's breathing became and how frequently she had to stop, broke into tears. She cried and said, "I don't like it. I don't like being afraid of losing you. I don't know what I'd do without you."

Henrietta replied, "This is what happens in life when you love. If you are so afraid of losing, you can't see the life that is here."

"Then it was over," she told me. "It was OK, and it was just a happy, happy day."

My patient cried as she told me this story. I knew how physically active she used to be and how hard it was for her now to go slowly. She had not wanted her daughter to discover that her condition had worsened. Neither she nor her daughter was reconciled to this change. This attitude shifted a few weeks later after Henrietta discovered that a good friend of hers, who also had congestive heart failure, had died. He had ignored his symptoms and denied their gravity, failing to take his medication regularly. She realized that she, like him, would die prematurely if she continued to "fake it" and keep pretending she was fine. By trying to protect her daughter, she realized she was harming herself and damaging their relationship by blocking honest communication. This delayed both of them from accepting her disabilities.

Conditions can worsen at any time, and we live with this knowledge. Our "normal" has changed. Adaptation requires flexibility, resilience, and honesty. Denial perpetuates fear and prolongs suffering.

· · · · · · · · · ·

STOP

What losses are you aware of? What is your process of acceptance?

· · · · · · · · · ·

When my mother had a massive stroke and was unconscious, my father called me to come home. I lived in another city, and I could not arrive immediately. When I got there, I found him on the floor next to where she lay. He had spent the night with her. At the time, I was horrified, but later (much later) I understood that it was his way of saying good-bye. My mother, as we knew her, was gone and would never return. My father understood nothing could be done, so he did what was meaningful to him and lay beside her until the inevitable ambulance ride to the hospital. This was autumn, and during the two weeks before she died, he brought colorful leaves that had fallen from the trees and pinned them to the bulletin board on her wall. Later, as part of my grieving process, I, too, picked up some bright leaves from the ground. Thinking I could preserve their color, I dipped them in paraffin and incorporated them into a watercolor I was painting. I carefully framed the picture and hung it in my house. In time, the leaves dried and the colors faded, but it stills hangs where I can see it, a reminder that everything passes, but love remains.

It is not easy to truly let go and be accepting of change, but when we do, it is so freeing that we may wonder why it took so long. Our tendency is to fear the unknown. Something bad but familiar can feel more comfortable than entering a new place. Our ability to have faith and be trusting varies. We need to know that if we take the leap and let go, we will arrive at a safe place.

When I was on retreat several years ago, I heard a story that illustrates this point. A man is being chased by a tiger. The man is a fast runner and is slightly ahead of the tiger, but he comes to a cliff and has to halt. There is a sheer drop below and no handholds to navigate down. He cannot go forward, and the tiger is waiting to eat him if he tries to go back. Seeing the root of a tree growing on the side of the cliff, he grabs onto it and yells, "Help, help!"

A voice from the sky answers, "Yes?"

"What should I do?" the man cries out. "Save me."

"Let go, you will be released," the voice responds.

And the man says, "Anyone else out there?"

In a different version of the story, a rat begins gnawing away at the root. Rather than asking for help, the man spies a strawberry growing next to him and, with his free hand, reaches out to pick it and puts it in his mouth. Savoring its juiciness, he says, "Delicious."

. . . .

STOP

How do we react when we are backed up against the wall and there is no way out? Do we refuse to accept our situation, or can we see a strawberry, reach for it, and appreciate how juicy and delicious it is? What are our metaphorical strawberries?

. . . .

It is impossible not to have some regrets about what may or may not have happened in your life. Sometimes these can be repaired. I was teaching meditation to an experienced nurse who was new to hospice work but had lived with and cared for a disabled sister until her death. She was upset because the hospital had released a very sick patient into her care only six hours before he died. While she was meditating with me, she realized those few hours had been meaningful.

"Maybe I learned a thing or two," she told me, describing how she had urged one of the man's daughters, who had been estranged from him for many years, to move from the far side of the room and come and lie next to her father in the bed.

"It gave her closure," she said. "Her dad was in a coma. It was clear that she wanted to connect but didn't know how. I helped the family. There was much more peace when he passed."

We are all tender and vulnerable and can be ultrasensitive, especially when we are sick. This can create misunderstandings and strain communication. As we change, the people around us are also affected, and they change too. A long-lasting or chronic illness can deplete resources and wear down resilience. A once-patient caregiver can become irritable and vice versa. Parents worry about their children, and the children can be fearful, lacking the words to express their worries. They may act out nonverbally or become too quiet and overly compliant. Adults, too, have difficulty putting voice to what they feel and tolerating emotional volatility. Watching a loved one decline is disturbing. There is increased responsibility for the caregiver, and the relationship is changed and often strained.

Loss can be cumulative or sudden. A single young woman who has had a breast removed may be self-conscious and afraid to date. Chemotherapy can induce premature menopause. Prostrate cancer can take away sexual function and decrease virility. Sexual desire can wane, and we may think of ourselves as less sexual beings. Fatigue can be disabling and take the zest out of life. The body is less predictable. We may be more subject to injury or lose a bodily function. We may no longer be able to ambulate or even feed ourselves. Anything can happen at any time. With cancer, unlike a cold, we have no confidence that this will pass, and we will return to "normal." There is a new normal now. It is unfamiliar and can feel alien.

Friendships change, and we may be out of sync with loved ones.

When I was first diagnosed, I was too much in shock to feel much emotion; my husband cried and I comforted him. Later, as the seriousness of my illness became clear and my daily activities were altered, I had trouble adapting to this new reality, while he had more equanimity. As my illness progressed, each change brought a new adjustment in our relationship to the illness and to each other. We needed to talk about end-of-life issues rather than waiting for a crisis. We had lengthy discussions about where we would be buried. I refused to be buried in Worcester, where I have no family and the cemetery is ugly, but years ago, we had bought a plot there because convenience is primary for my husband. I think family and aesthetics are important. After lengthy discussions, we agreed to use my parents' plot in New York. The only problem is that there are four slots, and my father chose a middle position for himself and my mother, thinking my brother and I would be buried on either side of them. My brother has chosen cremation, which leaves my husband, David, next to one parent and me next to the other. We joke about which side we'll choose. Should he be next to my mother in the earth, or could we be on top of each other? A more serious discussion is when to pull the plug. This is more complicated and an ongoing contemplation.

I see many patients who are ill or have sick family members who are grieving. I feel their grief and need to remind myself (and others) of the power of witnessing strong feelings and providing a safe space for them to be expressed. It is easy to feel helpless and not acknowledge the strength it takes to be with another who is suffering. Our own fear and loss can interfere with our ability to be wholly with them. Simply sitting next to a loved one, breathing in rhythm with her breath, holding her hand, listening, and silently expressing love is potent and a deep connection. We are fortunate if we can grieve.

Hearts break open out of love. It is a gift to care and a blessing to share loss as well as joy.

. . . .

May we all be free of suffering.

. . . .

Meditation

I suggest you do this at a time when you will not be interrupted and in an environment that feels safe and protected. Do your best to come into a position of receptivity and comfort that is supportive. If you are lying down, you can spread your feet a few inches apart and have your arms resting alongside your body, palms facing upward. If you are sitting, let the position also be one of relaxed awareness, open and supportive. You may open your palms and let your arms rest on the body or chair. Let your eyes close or choose a point in front of you. Allow your eyes to focus on it until you feel your eyelids getting heavy and closing.

Allowing your breathing to come into a relaxed rhythm, bring your attention into your body and sweep through it with loving attention, softening into and lingering at any spot that seems to require some extra care. Taking a deep breath in, and deepening your relaxation, let yourself rest here, allowing an image of vastness and spaciousness to emerge. You might picture yourself lying at the beach, letting yourself be supported and sinking into the warmth and solidity of the soft sand. As you breathe in, perhaps you can smell the saltiness of the air and feel the coolness of a breeze touching you lightly and tenderly, refreshing and healing. You may feel the warmth of the sunlight and the texture of the sand, helping you relax and be at ease. Let this ease deepen as you hear the sounds around you, the roar of the waves meeting the shore, the voices of people, or the songs of the birds. Perhaps you are in a beautiful meadow or some other lovely spot, sitting in a favorite chair or lying on your back and viewing the sky and all that passes by. You can notice how it changes, the colors filling its space, and any clouds or shapes that enter your vision.

As you breathe in, soften into any sense that blocks the heart and obstructs your vision. Feel the release of air and any heaviness or darkness that needs liberation, sending it out into the vastness and spaciousness present here. Let yourself be surrounded by the cocoon of love that envelops and protects you. You can repeat words of loving-kindness and compassion to yourself, following my suggestions or your own.

May I connect to the universality of life.
May I feel the vastness of time and space.
May I feel my connection to the world around me,
the people I know and love and all that exists.
May I know the universality of caring.
May I be held in the womb of love.
May I be blessed and protected.
May my wounds heal.
May heaviness and darkness pass like clouds in the sky.
May I forgive my errors and know the compassion of forgive-
ness.
May I have faith in the good.
May I live with joy and peace.
May love flow through me and bring peace to all that is.

Bringing attention to the area of the heart and resting here in this moment, trust what arises as you give yourself this space and time to nurture yourself and bring compassion to what clouds the mind and closes the heart. Let yourself connect to the universality of love and the wisdom of life's lawfulness.

You can allow an image to emerge that is your own personal sanctuary, a refuge where you can be fully at ease and at rest, where you can mourn what is lost and be at peace with what is here, letting the river of sorrow flow out into the vastness of the sea. This may or may not happen, but the intention to soften into sorrow will help it flow and be transformed.

15 / Gratitude

Even after all this time,
The sun never says to the earth,
"You owe me."
Look what happens with
A love like that.
It lights the whole sky.
        —*Hafiz of Persia*

Each day, there are moments when I find myself internally saying, "Thank you." It happened today as I went off to teach. I am in another city, and I am grateful for the opportunity to share this work with others. I am thankful I have the energy to get myself there. Driving to the airport, I turned off the news, enjoyed the quiet, and appreciated that the traffic continued to move even though it was rush hour and the day after a holiday weekend. I mentally noted gratitude as I maneuvered my way through crowds and pulled my heavy suitcase laden with books. I was aware of the effort it took to wheel it to the check-in counter and grateful to see the conveyor belt take it off my hands. As I continued through security and walked down the long corridor to the gate with my tote bag, laptop, and miscellaneous "necessities," I noted the sensation of heaviness and appreciated that

I was strong enough to go on the trip. Having the stamina to travel is a gift. I do not take it for granted.

Sometimes gratitude overtakes me. I feel it radiating from my heart up into my head and down into my body. In those moments, I am fully content. It is not excitement but a deep appreciation that my senses register. There is a sense of completeness and peace. Wanting ceases, and I am content.

I wasn't always like this. Not being able to perform natural functions woke me up to the miracle of my daily life and routine activities. I remember how proud and grateful I was in the hospital to roll my IV into the bathroom, hold on to the rail, and balance myself to use the facility. It was a gift when my immune system recovered sufficiently for a nurse to wheel me outdoors. I remember sitting in my wheelchair, the wonder of breathing unfiltered air, and the miracle of feeling it on my cheek.

There are so many things to be grateful for. I am grateful that I have been able to celebrate being married for twenty-five years, and my husband and I make the effort to notice the small things and express appreciation to each other. He has taught me to say, "Thank you." "Thank you for bringing me a cup of tea"; "Thank you for going with me to this event"; "Thank you for washing the dishes"; "Thank you for living with my foibles."

As I have learned to appreciate the simple courtesies of life in relation to him and others, I have also learned to appreciate myself and my own efforts to be kind and caring. Instinctively, we all yearn for love and reach for warmth and comfort. Sometimes we get it; at other times, we don't. When I was young and needed comfort, I needed to learn to comfort myself. Nesting deeply in my bed and swaddling myself with blankets, my arm around my pillow, I would say a prayer I had learned in kindergarten. It was the only prayer I knew by heart:

Thank you, God, for the world so sweet,
Thank you, God, for the food I eat,
Thank you, God, for the birds that sing,
Thank you, God, for everything.

Giving thanks soothed me. It took me outside myself and refocused my attention. The part of me that was scared disappeared. I was ten and unprepared to face old age and death. My mother's parents, whom we were hoping to help, had come to live with us, and we had moved to accommodate them. Bubbe and Zaydie (Yiddish for Grandma and Grandpa) were old and sick and spoke a foreign language. I didn't know they had dementia or Alzheimer's, and their erratic behavior scared me. It seemed the whole household was upset and disconnected.

This was almost sixty years ago, but my memory of comforting myself with this prayer remains reassuring. Somehow, everything is all right. The world is sweet. There are birds that sing. I can eat. There is food. I am alive. I feel secure and protected. Gratitude overrides fear and confusion, and I calm.

I am grateful for connection, understanding, warmth, and caring. My cousin Luba, who is in her seventies, is now undergoing treatment for lymphoma. She has recently adjusted to the death of her husband of fifty-four years, who died of leukemia a few years ago. She has learned to be independent, but her relationships with friends and family enrich and support her. "They are wonderful," she tells me—and also them.

Luba was nauseous when I last saw her, but she did not complain. She was able to laugh, tell stories, and tell us how lucky she felt between bouts of sickness.

"I like my life," she said. "Whatever happens, I'll be all right. There is much to celebrate."

I met Svein Myreng at Plum Village, a retreat center in the south of France created by Vietnamese monk Thich Nhat Hahn to heal broken hearts ravaged by war. Svein was a quiet, soft-spoken, slim young man from Denmark. He had been born with a life-threatening heart condition. His physical heart was broken, but his emotional/spiritual heart was whole. There was a stillness and thoughtfulness about him that drew me to him. His condition seemed to bring out a sweetness in him that allowed him to savor every moment. Svein died in the late nineties, but his poems survive. In 1993, he wrote,

Celebration

I want to celebrate chaos.
I want to celebrate old worn-out cars,
Broken tiles, ever-shifting
Schedules, misplaced letters,
And nettles next to flowerbeds;
To celebrate toilets out of order,
As well as friends who will remind me
That mistakes are good, failure a success,
And that a pure heart may prevail
In the non-end.
I want to celebrate being left alone,
or assailed by talkers,
(or, disturbing others' quiet).

I want to celebrate gentle smiles,
Good intentions, and, especially,
One step after the other.
"If arrow number 100 hits the target,
how can you say the first 99 were failures?"*

Svein knew the gift of placing one foot in front of the other and connecting to the earth. He was grateful for each step taken. Knowing each breath could be his last heightened his appreciation of what we might consider annoying or so ordinary that we would be blind to the wonder of its existence.

Can we honor our mistakes and be grateful that they are part of our being human? Life is so much more (and less) than our minds can fathom. Can we celebrate the humanness that allows us to grow and change, live and die? What are we bequeathing to our children and the generations to follow? Life is wild and chaotic. Change is a constant. Can gratitude follow even in the midst of sickness and pain? When I posed this question to my brother, Bob, a neuropsychologist, he told me about a patient of his who knew she had the gene for Huntington's disease. Huntington's is hereditary and causes dementia. It is usually dormant until one reaches one's fifties. Once it starts, it advances rapidly. This is dramatic and disturbing to both patient and family. Several years ago, Bob established his patient's baseline and has been monitoring her for changes that would signal the onset of the disease. She is now in her fifties, and upon testing, he recently found early signs of the disease. This upset him, and in giving the patient the news, he prefaced his findings by saying, "I'm sorry."

---

* Svein Myreng, *Plum Poems* (Berkeley, CA: Parallax Press, 1998).

"Why are you sorry?" she asked him.

"I feel bad. You have the early signs of dementia; it has begun."

"Don't be sorry for me," she told him. "I am so grateful that I have had the gift of knowing that I have this. I've enjoyed every moment of my life, and now I know I really don't have much time, so I will be very careful about being with my family and loving my kids and enjoying and appreciating every minute of my life. Don't feel sorry for me. It's others I feel sorry for. They do not know when they will die, and they are missing their lives."

None of us knows when we will die or how old we will grow to be. We do know how we are living our lives. Each moment does count. May we enter into it with gratitude and love.

May we be well and live in harmony and peace.

A Guided Meditation: Gratitude

Finding a position that allows your body to be awake, supported, and comfortable, let your attention rest in the heart center and allow your imagination to fill it with light. Enveloping it in luminosity and love, let yourself receive whatever fills your heart with gratitude. Take your time. Don't try to make anything happen. Simply note the nature of what arises. What is its form? Are there colors and shapes? Can you feel sensations in the body along with thoughts and feelings?

Give yourself the time and space to explore what does or does not emerge, without an agenda, with permission to receive what is here for you. Let whatever is present be met and noted with gratitude for what it is telling you. Perhaps you will note temperature changes. You may feel heat or cold, the warmth of love or the coolness of ease. Let the light surrounding your heart deepen and penetrate your being.

With each breath, meeting what arises with tenderness and love, let the light of your attention shine with compassion into any part of you that is vulnerable. Notice how it changes. Breathing in and out through the region of the heart, you can thank it for taking care of you and helping you reach this moment. Letting your awareness fill with gratitude, soften into the moment, receptive and open to knowing and appreciating this moment and the presents that are within and without.

When there is a sense of completeness, you can return your attention to the breath, remembering your intention to be well and appreciating your ability to appreciate the wonders around you and inside you that are caring and expansive.

. . . .

EXERCISE: MY GRATITUDE LIST

Please fill in the blanks:

I am grateful for _____

I am grateful for _____

I am grateful for _____

I am grateful for _____

. . . .

16 / Enough

Sometimes we are so filled with love and gratitude that we are suffused with peace. We are satisfied. There is nothing more we want or crave. It is enough; we are content. How wonderful to live and die with this sense of completeness. How wonderful to be understanding and forgiving when all feels right in our world.

There are other times when we've had "enough," and our cup is overflowing not with peace, but with anger, fear, or desire. This, too, is profound. It can be a moment of awakening rather than resistance, a reminder to STOP and remember how we want to live and die.

In writing this book, I am aware of how much I have wanted to give you "enough" to realize your own strength and help you know that you are whole and have "enough" to be well, even while sick. As long as we are breathing and have the mental acuity to be aware of the workings of our mind/heart, there is always something to learn and to know. We can say, "Enough," and stop struggling to change what is unchangeable. With compassion, we can investigate the cause of our suffering and respond constructively. This can range from making the difficult decision to stop treatment and accept that everything has an end, including ourselves, to ending habits that no longer serve us. Then we can open to love and compassion and connect to what heals. Every time we note that our attention is in the past or future and redirect our attention to the present, we are silently demonstrating our power to affect the way we live. This takes courage and practice.

In summation:

1. Believe in the possible, but base it on the truth of the moment.
2. Remember that everything changes.
3. Practice kindness.
4. Connect to what is dear to you.
5. Soften into the moment.
6. Go bigger, look out, let be, and let in love.

Everything does have an ending, be it our life or this book. The meditations, exercises, and thoughts here are intended to be used repeatedly, examined, and questioned so that they have meaning for you. Wellness is yours right now. This moment is precious, as are you. Accepting it brings healing, and with it, peace.